Understanding the Effects of Concussion, Blast & Brain Injuries

A Guide for Families, Veterans, Service Members and Caregivers

Lash & Associates Publishing/Training Inc.

ISBN 978-1-931117-43-2

9 781931 117432

Cover Photo By:
Dan Conover/xark.typepad.com

Field of flags/eye level.
Each of these flagpoles includes a yellow ribbon that bears the name of an
American killed in our ongoing wars.

The "healing field" at Marion Square, Charleston, SC
www.healingfield.org

Library of Congress Control Number: 2007939786

Published by Lash & Associates Publishing/Training Inc.
708 Young Forest Drive, Wake Forest, NC 27587
Tel: & Fax: (919) 562-0015

This book is part of a series on brain injury among children, adolescents and adults.
For a free catalog, contact Lash & Associates
Tel. & Fax (919) 562-0015 or visit our website *www.lapublishing.com*

Lash & Associates Publishing/Training Inc.

708 Young Forest Drive, Wake Forest, North Carolina 27587-9040

Table of Contents

Articles on Behavior and Cognition

Articles on Life in the Community

Articles on College and Working

Introduction

Written by: Marilyn Lash MSW; Senior Editor; Lash & Associates Publishing/Training Inc.

Why this guide was written

This guide has been written to help the families of service members who have sustained traumatic brain injuries. It is also intended for the caregivers, clinicians and therapists who work with them over the various stages of their treatment and recovery. Traumatic brain injury has become known as the signature wound of the war in Iraq and conflicts in Afghanistan. While helmets, protective body gear and armored vehicles help protect troops during combat and on patrol, they still are exposed to possible injury or death each day that they are in a war zone. The sophisticated battlefield medicine and rapid air transport that are provided when a service member is injured have resulted in extraordinarily high rates of survival among the troops who have been injured. Unfortunately, some have not survived and their deaths are tragic losses for their families and this country.

Service members with traumatic brain injuries

The global war on terror is resulting in new types of traumatic injuries. In previous conflicts, troops fought on the front lines of combat. There is no "front line" in Iraq and Afghanistan. The war is being fought in local neighborhoods, open markets, cafes and routine traffic stops. Sniper fire, explosions and ambushes are part of daily life for support, transport and combat troops. This lack of a safety zone creates additional stresses and risks for troops who must be on alert 24 hours a day, 7 days a week. Extended and multiple deployments add to the emotional stress and physical risks. Shock waves and blasts from improvised explosive devices (IEDs), land mines and rocket propelled grenades can cause terrible damage to the human body. Many service members have had injuries to multiple body areas – called polytrauma in medical terms. They are returning to the US with missing limbs, the scars of painful burns, and loss of vision or hearing. The brain is especially vulnerable in an explosion, collision or fall as it is the most complex organ in the body – and it controls how we think, act, move, feel, and communicate.

Just the words "traumatic brain injury" raises all sorts of questions and images. No two brain injuries are alike. Consequently, the recovery of each individual with a brain injury is unique. A mild brain injury (often called a concussion) may have temporary effects that last for only several hours, days or weeks. However, multiple concussions can have more serious effects over time. Moderate to severe brain injuries can result in more serious damage and increase the likelihood that a service member will become disabled. A traumatic brain injury can result in visible physical changes. Some individuals literally have to learn how to walk, talk, communicate, and do the basics of daily life all over again.

Consequences of traumatic brain injury

It is the changes in a person's thinking, reasoning, behavior, and personality after a brain injury that are usually harder for others to understand. These are the less visible but major consequences of a traumatic brain injury that can have life long effects on an individual's life and the family. A brain injury can change how a service member thinks, remembers, reasons, organizes, plans and problem solves – the very abilities that are essential for independent and active lives. There are also psychological and social changes that can alter the personality so that the individual literally seems like a different person. Impulsive, explosive and unpredictable behaviors and actions can be the direct result of damage to certain areas of the brain. It is these changes in thinking, emotions and behavior that become the most challenging over time for families and caregivers as service members return to their homes and communities.

This guide will help the service members, their families and caregivers understand the immediate and long-term consequences of traumatic brain injury. Ironically, if a silver lining can be found, it is that today's veterans with brain injuries have the good fortune of timing. The medical treatment and rehabilitation of adults with traumatic brain injury has made many gains over the past 30 years. Brain injury medicine and rehabilitation has made amazing advances in care and treatment since the Vietnam War. That expertise is helping our service members injured in the Global War on Terror. We are now learning about the new types of brain injuries caused by blast injuries and shock waves and are using state of the art medicine. We also know from the struggles of previous veterans that post traumatic stress disorder (PTSD) can have serious consequences if unidentified and untreated. We have learned from the past. The advances in brain injury treatment are helping our service members who are being treated in the polytrauma centers under the Department of Defense, the Veterans Administration Hospitals and Clinics, and within the private civilian sector.

Coming home

The next big challenge for many service members comes when they return home. Surviving a brain injury is one thing; living with a brain injury is another. The transition from living in a war zone to coming home is not always a smooth nor easy one. Life has changed. Children have been born and grown, couples have grown together or split apart, roles and responsibilities have shifted, jobs have changed, homes have moved. This transition will be even more stressful and complicated for the family with a service member who is coming home with a traumatic brain injury. Programs and services in local communities for survivors of traumatic brain injuries and their families have not grown at the same pace as medical and rehabilitation services. Just sorting out the disability and health benefits and coverage under the various programs for active duty military, veterans and reservists is a challenge. The community of individuals and families living with brain injury stretches far and wide. Unfortunately, it continues to grow. While each person and each family are unique, the experience of having one's life changed by an injury to the brain unites them.

How to use this guide

This guide will help readers understand the many dimensions of traumatic brain injury. It provides tips and strategies for coping and moving forward as service members and their families resume and rebuild their lives. It gives an overview of the many dimensions of brain injury with more in-depth detail on specific topics. Many of he articles were originally published by Lash and Associates Publishing/Training Inc. as "Tip Cards" on specific aspects of brain injury and were written by experts in the field of traumatic brain injury. This tip card format was chosen because families and caregivers said they needed information they could quickly read and absorb that was written in clear language with prac-

tical suggestions or tips on what to look for, what to do and strategies to use. This format and style has been used again for this guide because it provides a quick summary with action steps without all the jargon. We have chosen all the tip cards that are relevant for service members, their families and caregivers. They have been revised and made into a collection of articles for this guide.

Not all the articles will apply to all individuals, their families or caregivers. Readers are encouraged to pick and choose the sections and articles that fit your situation. As the person progresses and recovers, topics of interest and needs for information will change. That is why we have put all the information together in this guide. It is a resource that you can go back to repeatedly over time as new questions, challenges and needs emerge. There is literally something for everyone in this guide.

Section 1 – Articles on Helping Families

Just as life changed for you when your family member went to war, it has changed again with the diagnosis of a brain injury. Families have many worries, fears, questions and uncertainties as they face the future after a loved one has been injured. Once the immediate danger of whether the person will survive has passed, the question becomes, "What will she be like? Will he be different now? How will our family manage?" Whether it is your son or daughter, brother or sister, husband or wife, cousin, aunt or uncle – the entire family is affected by a brain injury.

This section has articles to help families cope during the initial days, weeks or months of hospital care and rehabilitation. It discusses changes in the relationship between spouses or partners after the service member comes home as responsibilities change and daily life is reorganized. Suggestions for talking to children when a parent has a brain injury are given with considerations for the child's age and understanding.

The power of emotions and methods for coping are discussed as families come to realize that life may never be the same again. Warning signs of stress and depression among caregivers as well as the individual with a brain injury are described. As roles and responsibilities shift and family members become caregivers, balancing the needs of everyone while holding the family together can feel like a juggling act with no breather. Suggestions are given to avoid caregiver stress and burnout and methods for becoming efficient coordinators for services and care.

Section 2 - Articles on Concussion and Trauma

The severity of a brain injury can range from mild to severe. Even a mild brain injury or a concussion can have consequences. For those with more severe brain injuries, the period of coma can be frightening and stressful. This section contains two articles on coma and concussion to help families recognize symptoms and monitor recovery.

Post traumatic headache and post traumatic stress disorder can slow and complicate a service member's recovery and make it harder to function at home, back at work, and in the community. They may affect the service member's ability to return to duty. They are described in detail with suggestions on how and when to seek help.

Section 3 - Articles on Medications

This section goes into detail about the use of medications after brain injury and how they work. It is a useful resource for families to use to discuss concerns and questions about medications with physicians who may be prescribing drugs and monitoring their effects.

Section 4 - Articles on Behavior and Cognition (thinking)

Changes in a service member's behavior, thinking, learning, personality, communication, social skills, memory, and self awareness can be the most difficult changes for family members. The brain does not heal like a broken bone. It is commonly said that, "War changes a person." So does a brain injury. The combination of being in combat and having a brain injury is powerful. It can affect a service member in more ways than physical injuries. Many families report that their loved one seems like a new person – and this makes it hard to know what to expect and how to respond. This section explains why a person may act and think differently after a brain injury and gives many practical tips for families and caregivers on how to help.

Section 5 - Articles on Life in the Community

Recovery from a moderate or severe brain injury can be a long journey. As service members who have survived a brain injury try to pick up their lives at home and in the community, families often worry about how much help, support or assistance is needed. This section provides a checklist for families and caregivers to guide them as they consider what is needed for the person's safety, independence and supervision.

The use of alcohol poses special risks for anyone who has had a brain injury. These risks are explained with suggestions for finding treatment programs and getting help for substance abuse.

There is even an article about concerns for aging after a person has a brain injury. While many of our military are now young, we all grow older each year. For other service members now in mid life, these concerns may be more pressing.

Section 6 - Articles on College and Working

Life after military service involves decisions about college, vocational training, and employment. An individual with a brain injury may need accommodations on the job or may need retraining or schooling to find a new job. This section gives information about vocational resources and programs in the states as well as federal laws that protect workers with a disability from discrimination.

Section 7 - Resources

Developing this section was difficult because the military and civilian sectors are very different.

Just navigating the complex system of health care and benefits for various branches of the service and national guard is a challenge. This can be even more stressful when a family is dealing with the effects of a traumatic brain injury and the uncertainties of the future.

While many programs and agencies dedicated to supporting service members discussed post deployment adjustment, it was difficult to identify resources that addressed this for the service member who had had a traumatic brain injury. On the other hand, there are many programs and services in the civilian sector with expertise in traumatic brain injury, but they may have little knowledge of, or experience with, service members. There is also the challenge of figuring out eligibility under the Veterans Administration, TRICARE, Social Security, private insurance and state services. The resources described in this section provide a starting point for understanding this complex system.

Frequently Asked Questions about Traumatic Brain Injury

What is a traumatic brain injury?

The brain is the organ in the body that controls how we move, think, act and feel. An injury to the brain can have many different effects on a person. The consequences of an injury depend on what areas of the brain are hurt and how severely they are damaged. The term "traumatic brain injury" is used because it is an injury that is caused by an external force or trauma.

Among civilians, the most common causes of traumatic brain injury are car crashes, falls, assaults, and sports injuries. Examples of trauma are the person's head hitting the windshield in a car crash, the face being beaten in a fight, or a heavy hit and fall to the ground in a football game.

The soft tissue of the brain is protected inside the head's hard bony skull. But when a person's head hits something hard such as the ground or pavement, the brain can move around inside the skull from the force of the impact. This movement can cause bleeding, bruising, tearing and swelling in the brain. Brain cells can literally be torn apart. The brain can also be injured without the head being struck directly. This can happen with a whiplash injury.

No two traumatic brain injuries are alike. The effects of a traumatic brain injury are different for each person.

Why are troops and service members at risk for a traumatic brain injury?

Service members are exposed to many risks for a traumatic brain injury. Combat is the most obvious danger where bullets, shrapnel or debris can penetrate the skull and enter the brain. The blasts and explosions from improvised explosive devices, rocket propelled grenades and land mines in Iraq and Afghanistan have resulted in many traumatic brain injuries among troops and support personnel.

Combat is not the only risky arena. Crashes or collisions of helicopters, tanks, trucks, and other vehicles have resulted in traumatic brain injuries to service members during training, transport and deployment. Falls are another major cause.

What is a blast injury?

The change in air pressure caused by the blast can send shock waves through the brain and damage the very soft brain tissue. Debris from the blast can penetrate the brain. The force of the blast can throw a person to the ground, against a wall or other hard surfaces. The impact of the blast and the collision may result in a traumatic brain injury. If the person stops breathing, for even a short time, the flow of oxygen to the brain may be interrupted and cause a condition called anoxia. Poisonous chemicals or materials exposed by the blast can also damage the brain.

How is a brain injury treated?

Any type of brain injury needs immediate treatment. Most severe brain injuries are recognizable because of noticeable damage around the head or a loss of consciousness. However, less severe brain injures may not be as obvious, especially when attention is focused on multiple injuries to the body or other conditions that are life threatening for the individual. This can occur in cases of spinal cord injury, amputation, severe systemic injury, internal injuries or other major physical damage.

Does the person have to lose consciousness?

A person can have a brain injury without losing consciousness. These are called "mild" brain injuries, but they can have serious effects. A service member may feel dazed or confused after an explosion or collision and try to "shake it off". A service member who is briefly knocked out and then regains consciousness and resumes action may not realize what has happened. The majority of brain injuries fall into the "mild" category with temporary symptoms although a small number of people will have effects over longer periods of time.

A series of repeated hits, falls, crashes or blasts can have combined or cumulative effects over time and increase the chances of damage to the brain. The effects of these repeated injuries are being recognized among football players, prizefighters and other athletes involved in contact sports. A service member's exposure to repeated blasts increases the risk of an unidentified mild brain injury. Failure to recognize the symptoms of a concussion or mild brain injury can expose a service member to further risk in combat if concentration, alertness and responses are affected. Sometimes a concussion or mild brain injury is not recognized immediately because a service member is evacuated for life threatening injuries requiring immediate surgery and intensive care.

Is it ever too late to treat a brain injury?

No, it is never too late. A diagnosis may actually be a relief because it can explain why a person is feeling "not like myself" or having unexplained difficulties. The effects of a brain injury are not always recognized right away. Sometimes changes in a service member's behavior, emotions or thinking are thought to be due to combat fatigue, stress or nerves. The effects of a brain injury can be subtle and require careful screening by a neurologist, neuropsychologist or other brain injury expert. This is why many Veterans Administration Hospitals and Clinics are conducting special screening tests to identify undiagnosed brain injury among returning soldiers.

What about PTSD?

Post traumatic stress disorder used to be referred to as "combat fatigue" among veterans of earlier wars. The long-term effects of untreated PTSD became tragically evident among many veterans of the Vietnam War. As service members return from conflicts in Iraq and Afghanistan, increased attention is being given to screening and treating symptoms of PTSD to help service members recover and resume their lives. PTSD is not a brain injury. But service members with brain injuries may also have PTSD.

Can someone recover from a severe brain injury?

It is impossible to precisely predict how anyone will recover from a more serious brain injury because there are so many factors to consider. However, service members injured in the Middle East conflicts have the highest rates of survival of any war involving US troops. This is directly due to advances in battlefield medicine and the quick evacuation and transport of injured troops to specialized trauma centers.

Service members with serious brain injuries face the same fundamental questions as civilians with brain injuries. How will this affect my life, my family and my future? The pattern and extent of recovery will differ for each person.

How are families affected?

From the day that their spouses, parents, sons, daughters, brothers or sisters were deployed, families have worried about their safety and waited for their safe return home. Whether loved ones are in direct combat or serving as support personnel, they are still in a dangerous place and away from home. Children are missing parents, spouses are living without mates, and future plans are put on hold. Days, weeks and months are counted until loved ones come home safely.

The news that your loved one has been injured brings fear, stress and uncertainty for the family. The initial reaction is the relief that comes with survival. Then the questions become... What is a traumatic brain injury? Will he recover? Will she be different? and How will this affect our lives? This guide will help you and your family as you try to answer those questions.

Life after Brain Injury
A Guide for Families
Written by: Carolyn Rocchio, Parent & Marilyn Lash, M.S.W.

✓ describes emotions of families
✓ identifies changes at home
✓ gives community resources
✓ discusses long-term issues

Emotional Reactions

Shock, fright and bewilderment are common reactions during the medical and emotional crisis of brain injury.

You may be feeling

- a roller coaster of emotions
- drained and overwhelmed with responsibility
- alone and isolated from everything familiar
- angry that a member of your family was injured
- guilty that you were unable to prevent the injury.

You may be worried about

- costs of treatment and rehabilitation
- time off from work
- your family member's recovery
- reactions of others in the family
- the financial impact on your family.

Just when you most need to talk about your feelings, others may not understand what you are going through. The optimism or assurances of friends may sound false and remind you of how much is still unknown about your family member's brain injury. As you turn to professionals for information and assurance, you will find that their ability to explain medical terms and procedures clearly varies, as do their attitudes and availability.

Coping with the Hospital Stay

Tips for gathering information in the hospital...

✓ Choose a family member to gather and write down information.
✓ Make a written list of names and telephone numbers of doctors, nurses, therapists, specialists, and others.
✓ Start a journal to record progress over time.
✓ Write down how you feel each day.
✓ Request copies of medical records and/or the discharge summary. Never give up your set. Make copies for others who need this information.

Tips for gathering information about brain injury...

✓ Contact the Brain Injury Association of America's Family Help line at 1-800-444-6443 or go to their web site at www.biausa.org
✓ Contact your state's Brain Injury Association.
✓ Talk to other families with similar experiences.
✓ Ask social workers, case managers or discharge planners for information on brain injury.
✓ Start a filing system for your information and records.
✓ Search the Internet by using key words of traumatic brain injury, blast injury, military service member and veteran.

Tips for emotional support...

✓ Let friends know how to help you and your family by
   - providing transportation if needed
   - bringing in meals
   - baby-sitting/checking on others at home
   - running errands
   - checking mail.

✓ Contact people of your faith or religion.

✓ Expect family members to react and cope differently.

✓ Arrange for respite or relief from your hospital visits.

✓ Take care of yourself, get sleep, and eat regularly.

✓ Join a support group. Many hospitals have them. Request a list from your state Brain Injury Association.

✓ If you are not ready now for a support group, try one later as your situation changes.

Moving to Rehabilitation
You may be feeling...

- worried about the effects of the move
- concerned about the experience of new staff
- reluctant to move your family member further away
- that this nightmare will never end and life will never be "normal" again
- uncertain what to expect regarding recovery
- chronically tired and frustrated by the long time away from your family, job and home.

Many families are surprised to find that...

- rehabilitation staff include them in therapy and instruction
- their family member seems less fragile once the medical crises have passed
- meeting families in similar situations leads to sharing information and networking
- they become more confident as caregivers
- they are less apprehensive about the future
- discharge planning renews hopes.

Going Home

Families eventually become the managers of care and services. Families know the person best and have an important role in designing effective and practical discharge plans, setting future goals and developing support systems.

Reentering the community

Going home can be challenging. Families often feel...

- disconnected from medical and rehabilitation staff
- isolated at home
- confused by the changes in their family member
- unable to think about the future
- disappointed when expectations of dramatic improvement once home fall short
- saddened when remembering how life used to be
- frustrated by comments about being overprotective
- worried about reactions of friends, classmates, relatives or coworkers
- concerned about the limited knowledge and experience of schools and employers about brain injury.

Tips for finding resources in the community...

A brain injury may occur at any stage of life. It can interrupt pursuing current plans and dreams for the future. It can disrupt family life in many ways. Expectations for recovery are different for each person. Many will need help to pursue higher education, enter or reenter employment, or return to homemaking and childrearing.

There are federal and state laws governing the rights of persons with disabilities. It is important to use them to find resources in the community.

Contacts in Your State or Community

All public colleges and universities have centers or offices for students with special needs. They can help arrange for a variety of accommodations or tutoring.

Every state has a vocational program for helping persons entering or reentering employment after an injury or illness results in special needs or a disability. The Department of Vocational Rehabilitation (different name in some states) can provide vocational assessments, testing, training, help on the job, and other services to help people become employed.

Community mental health programs can help with addiction disorders and psychological issues.

The Americans with Disabilities Act (ADA) is a federal law which requires that people with disabilities have equal opportunities in employment, housing, transportation, governmental services and telecommunications.

Every state has a Protection and Advocacy System. These agencies provide advocacy services for people who are disabled due to mental illness. These programs recently have been expanded to include people with traumatic brain injury.

States also have Client Assistance Programs which provide advocacy services to clients of state vocational rehabilitaion agencies.

Social Security Administration can provide financial assistance to qualified adults. Two important programs are Supplemental Security Income (SSI) and Social Security Disability Insurance (SSDI). (Website www.ssa.gov or call 800-772-1213)

Many states have trust funds and other programs just for persons with brain injuries.

All states are required to maintain Centers for Independent Living (CIL) with varying services ranging from case management to skills building training.

Many federal, state and local government agencies provide access to transportation services for persons who are unable to drive.

Counties and cities are good resources for recreational activities and most provide special access to recreational venues for persons with disabilities.

Life Goes On and So Do You

A serious injury affects everyone in the family differently. Over time you can build a different but fulfilling life. Many families discover qualities that would not have surfaced were it not for the injury. The fragility and meaning of life become more real. Feelings of loss and periods of grieving may recur, even years later, and remind you of lost hopes and dreams.

Tips for coping with long term changes...
✓ Recognize your limits and realize you cannot fix everything.
✓ Adjust to what has changed and move on.
✓ Find activities in the community such as recreational programs, church/synagogue activities, youth programs, support groups, job clubs, social groups and military support groups.
✓ Pursue career goals.
✓ Return to and enjoy activities with other family members as before the injury.

Long term consequences

It is important for families to be alert for changes in mood and behavior as the individual improves over time. Some changes will be positive and lead toward greater independence. Other changes may be disruptive and signal the onset of difficulties requiring medical or psychological attention.

Increased awareness and insight into how life has changed may lead to the person with of a brain injury feeling more depressed, frustrated or angry. Professionals experienced in brain injury can help the individual and family develop strategies to compensate for difficulties with memory, attention, judgment, and reasoning. If family members continually reinforce these methods, the individual's difficulties may lessen and abilities may continue to grow. Changes in thinking and behavior after a brain injury often present the greatest challenge to the individual for fitting into the community and being accepted by others. It is wise to seek help early.

Some possible medical consequences requiring evaluation are:
- development of seizures months or years after the injury
- loss of bone density due to prolonged use of anti-convulsants
- endocrine disorders
- increased risk for Alzheimer's dementia
- visual changes

Persistent psychological consequences may include:
- anxiety and depressive disorders
- agitation/behavioral outbursts
- inappropriate behavior
- denial of deficits
- poor self-image

When you find positive ways to move on, your family member will move along with you. Brain injury doesn't go away. However, information and educational resources can better prepare families to negotiate the maze or complicated paths that define life in general after brain injury.

Recovery can extend over months and even years. There will be occasional wrong turns in the maze. Once a path through the maze is found, many survivors of brain injuries and their families find their lives have been enriched by the adversity. The reward is knowing that you have made a difference.

References

Rocchio, C. (1993). *Families as case managers.* TBI Challenge! Washington, DC: National Head Injury Association, Spring 1(2).

Rocchio, C. and Lash, M. (1998) *Helping Families Cope When a Child has a Brain Injury.* Wake Forest, NC: Lash & Associates Publishing/Training Inc.

Life Changes
When a Spouse or Partner has a Brain Injury
Written by: Janelle Breese Biagioni & Marilyn Lash, M.S.W.

✓ describes feelings of loss
✓ explains changes in roles
✓ recognizes importance of self-care
✓ shows how to set up a support system

Impact on the Family

A brain injury affects everyone in the family. Roles and responsibilities of the non-injured spouse/ partner*, and often those of their children, change very quickly. This can feel overwhelming. Some of the changes include...

- assisting with physical care
- giving emotional support
- supervising for safety
- helping with communication
- managing new behaviors
- advocating for legal, medical and community services
- supplementing, or solely providing family income.

*For simplicity, the word spouse is used for husband or wife; unmarried partners are also included.

Having lone responsibility for managing a home, including parenting and finances, can be incredibly stressful for the non-injured spouse. Common reactions are worrying, being confused, feeling overwhelmed, upset and frightened of the future. This can lead to anxiety, stress, anger and depression.

Loss is part of brain injury

Life has changed. For some, it will never be the same again. Others will eventually feel their lives are back to normal – or as close to it as may be possible now.

Some losses affect everyone in the family such as changes in finances, social life, and relationships. Others directly affect the spouse who has been injured, such as physical, emotional, and cognitive changes. The person with a brain injury may also lose a traditional position or identity within the family – as wage earner, disciplinarian, or homemaker. The other spouse feels the effects of these losses. But the most fundamental changes may be in the relationship between spouses.

These losses must be mourned and are part of grieving. Before one can take pleasure in life, one must first fully acknowledge and express the losses. Avoiding this can have long-term and devastating consequences. Allowing feelings of joy and happiness to emerge can be challenging. Laughter and cheerfulness are vital to our well-being. Yet, family members often feel guilty once they begin to enjoy life again, especially if they are not able to do so equally.

Importance of self-care

Many spouses are thrust into the role of caregiver, advocate, and primary parent. Many become the principle income earner. This often leaves the non-injured spouse with little or no time for one self. Changes in health care have also resulted in enormous amounts of patient care being handed over to families sooner as hospital and rehabilitation stays have shortened. A spouse may become consumed with getting a partner with a brain injury through the day and night. A caretaking spouse often does not take care of one's self. It's very important to recognize and reclaim the time needed to nurture one's body, mind and spirit.

Seeking professional help from a mental health professional is one way to care for and look after one's self. Talking with an expert can lead to a new perspective and more effective coping strategies. Good friends and support groups can also help. Obtaining outside help is not a sign of weakness, but a step toward support and guidance.

Tips for spouses and partners...

✓ Pay attention to nutrition to fuel your body; junk food is a quick fix that doesn't last.

✓ Take rest breaks to prevent physical exhaustion; small naps can help you catch-up and keep going.

✓ Talk with a trusted friend or advisor to relieve stress.

✓ Ask for help; be courageous, but delegate what you can to friends and family who want to help.

✓ Take time to acknowledge what you feel. There is no shame in crying. It is a healthy and safe way to express sorrow.

✓ Take time for yourself without feeling guilty. Keep involved in something besides caretaking to help you maintain your balance and perspective.

Activating a support system

Caring and advocating for a spouse is a lot of work and can be a full time job. It is easy to want to do it all, or to slip into trying to do it all without thinking about it. Family, friends and co-workers usually want to help, but may not know what to do. Assigning responsibilities such as shopping, cleaning, cooking, transporting children to school, sports and/or extra-curricular activities will give you a break. It offers a way for family and friends to support you. It's important to conserve your energy for daunting tasks like coordinating rehabilitation services, initiating legal action if necessary, and assisting in personal care. It's okay to ask for and accept help.

As you work through your emotions and feelings, it is critical to have ongoing support from family, friends, co-workers, and professionals in the community.

Tips for talking with children, family, friends and coworkers...

✓ Be as honest as you can.

✓ Don't withhold information.

✓ Inform others about good news as well as problems.

✓ Share the burden and the joys.

✓ Determine what needs to be done and delegate.

✓ Figure out what you need for yourself and ask for it.

✓ Ask for help from family and friends.

✓ Listen to your children and learn how the changes in your family are affecting them.

Parenting

Duties of parenting can quickly fall on the shoulders of the uninjured parent. This shift in responsibility can last for months and often years. The parent who has not been injured can feel besieged with double duties of caring for children and a spouse. With less time and attention from parents despite their best efforts, children can feel neglected and abandoned.

When possible, encourage your spouse to share some of the responsibilities of parenting. You may need to help your partner learn to do things again or learn to do them differently. Both the parent who has been injured and the child need ways and time to reconnect. Supervising younger children while they brush their teeth, or sitting with older children while they do homework are simple ways for the parent who has been injured to be involved. Identify fun things as well to improve the parent and child relationship.

Be patient and be supportive - adjusting takes time. It is important to remember that difficulties with concentration, understanding and frustration tolerance may affect a partner's ability to parent after an injury.

Children, like spouses, need to take care of themselves. Mini-vacations, exercise, hobbies, and entertainment are important. Teach them that they deserve to life their life fully and not feel guilty about it. LEAD BY EXAMPLE!

Tips for parenting...

✓ Ask for help if you need it.

✓ Solicit family and friends to give you a break so you can have one-on-one time with your child(ren).

✓ Ask other adults to help you so your child(ren) do not become burdened with duties beyond their age.

✓ Help children verbalize how they feel. At least one, but probably both parents have changed and children may find this hard to understand and adapt.

✓ Seek outside help from a professional or peer support group.

✓ Connect with other parents who share a similar situation.

✓ Find a support group for spouses through the Brain Injury Association in your state or province.

✓ Notify teachers about what has happened so they can give emotional support to your child and alert you to changes in behavior, grades or peer relationships.

✓ Keep communication open by acknowledging feelings and encouraging safe, appropriate expressions.

✓ Be prepared to do your own grief work and adapt.

✓ Don't be afraid to show your emotions and share your grief with your children. When possible, show them how you adapt and go on.

✓ Prepare younger children to cope with comments from peers who tell them that their parent walks or talks "funny" or acts "weird."

✓ Provide a safe, nurturing environment for teenagers who may be embarrassed by their parent's behavior or feel angry that life has changed so much. It's crucial not to judge; help them talk.

✓ Make communication among family members a priority.

Life Changes

It may be difficult to feel connected as a family after your spouse/partner returns home. It can be helpful to reflect on past traditions and routines of your family and find ways to do these customs and practices again. Some rituals may need to be altered. For example, if Dad usually reads a bedtime story but now has difficulty reading, perhaps Mom can read and Dad can sit and listen with the children. Other activities may need to go by the wayside or be scaled down to manageable events. For instance, if it is customary to entertain your entire extended family at holidays, consider inviting only a few.

Living as you did prior to the injury can give everyone a sense of security and routine in a time of stressful change. It's important to give yourselves time to settle into a new routine and to adjust to life now.

A person's view of the world can change after the crisis of brain injury. Family members may not feel like they belong anymore or they may show signs of insecurity. How they cope and interact with others can change over time. Families need to feel a sense of hope – something to show or make them feel that all will work out, that life is worth living and that some goodness will be restored.

Tips for reconnecting as a family...

✓ Reminisce about past events (look at photos or home videos and share stories).

✓ Enjoy the simple pleasures of short walks, fireside chats, or lingering at the dinner table.

✓ Have family meetings to discuss feelings, schedules, or to plan things as a family.

✓ Be patient! Everyone in the family may think their feelings are most important, but they may not be able to understand others during this challenging time.

✓ Try not to make any major decisions, i.e. selling the family home or moving to another city.

✓ Make sure that everybody has valued roles in the family, especially the spouse with the injury who may feel left out, devalued or a burden to others.

Intimacy

There are often disruptions in intimacy between couples after a partner has a brain injury. This is expected when the person is hospitalized, in a coma or living in a rehabilitation program. As the spouse recovers, emotional and physical intimacy may or may not return. Physical changes such as pain, sensitivity to touch, muscle incoordination, or poor stamina may present challenges for intimacy and sex.

Emotional and cognitive changes may make it difficult for the spouse who has been injured to anticipate the needs or desires of a mate. The spouse with a brain injury may no longer desire emotional or physical intimacy - or may demand it constantly. The caregiving husband or wife may not have the energy or desire - or may feel that their "new spouse" is a stranger due to changes in personality, emotions or physical appearance. A spouse who is a caretaker may not feel sexually attracted toward a partner who now needs to be bathed, toileted or fed. This is another loss.

Recovery can go on for months and years. The feelings of both spouses may change over time. Grief responses such as guilt, anger, sadness, confusion, frustration and loneliness can arise. Even the love between spouses may diminish or be questioned as the relationship changes.

Although difficult at times, it's important to accept how you feel. The first step in managing or controlling any feeling is to acknowledge it. Often just acknowledging a feeling reduces its intensity.

It's vital to identify and examine your feelings and then find ways to express and release them so you can move forward in your relationship.

Tips for reclaiming intimacy...

✓ Reflect on the intimacy you and your spouse/partner enjoyed prior to the brain injury. What changes are needed now and what are you comfortable with?

✓ Seek professional help for strategies, behavioral modifications and/or counseling if your spouse/partner is sexually/verbally inappropriate, lacks emotional sensitivity, or neglects personal hygiene.

✓ Ask relatives and friends to take your children overnight so you can create a quiet intimate space. This is very helpful when living on a limited budget.

✓ Be sure to get the rest you need. It's extremely hard to initiate intimacy, or to respond to it when you are exhausted.

✓ Enjoy intimate moments without expectations. Build upon a smile, soft touch, a shared laugh, or an embrace by lingering in the moment and allowing you and your partner to respond naturally.

✓ Explore new ways of sharing and pleasuring. Make this an adventure rather than a challenge.

Conclusion

Relationships are complex and constantly changing. Some become stronger; others dissolve and still others exist in a numbing emotional void. The stress of living with brain injury can challenge any couple and family. It is important for couples to grieve losses, adjust routines and responsibilities, find emotional support, and above all, communicate with each other in order to rebuild relationships after brain injury.

References

Breese Biagioni, J. (2004). *A Change of Mind: One Family's Journey through Brain Injury.* Wake Forest, NC: Lash and Associates Publishing/Training Inc.

Wolfelt, A. (1992). *Understanding Grief: Helping Yourself Heal.* Florence, KY: Accelerated Development.

Helping Sons and Daughters

When a Parent has a Brain Injury
Written by: Marilyn Lash, M.S.W. & Janelle Breese Biagioni

✓ describes the grieving process
✓ helps children cope
✓ prepares them for hospital visits
✓ prepares for changes at home

Life Changes Forever

Sons and daughters often say that, "No one else understood" what it was like after their parent's brain injury. They describe long days and nights of uncertainty, loneliness, and fear that a parent might die. With the joy and relief of a parent's survival comes uncertainty about the future.

Children of all ages need to grieve the loss of the known or idealized parent. Grief is not dependent on our ability to understand, but rather on our ability to feel. If a child has the capacity to love, the child has the capacity to mourn. Grief is a process – not an event. There is no time limit nor particular reactions or behaviors. Grieving will vary for each child and it can take many forms.

A brain injury can affect a parent's personality. The parent is still there but is different. The special parent/child relationship has been lost. The family as it was has been lost. This can be a death like experience for the child and family. The feelings of loss can be profound.

New responsibilities

The crisis of brain injury forces many children to grow up quickly – sometimes before they are ready. Some feel left out and forgotten at home; some feel overloaded with new responsibilities. Changes for children may be...

- helping with physical care
- giving emotional support
- supervising for safety
- helping with communication
- managing new behaviors
- supplementing income, and
- doing things that a parent used to do.

There may be no transition period for sons or daughters as they are thrust into an adult world with "adult worries." Many feel confused and upset and do not know what to do or how to ask for help. Some feel abandoned by relatives who are consumed by worries and stress.

Caring for younger siblings, preparing meals, doing laundry and going to school are often seen as reassuring signs of coping by relatives. Yet many children recall feeling confused, alone, angry and sad while they "did the things that needed to be done." Others felt they couldn't do things that were important to them like spending time with friends or after school activities.

Importance of communication

Many sons and daughters receive information about their parent's condition belatedly or second-hand by overhearing conversations in the hospital or at home. Many parents do not know how to explain what it means to have a brain injury. They are still struggling to understand what has happened and do not know what to expect next.

Caring adults may think that children are too young to understand and withhold information to protect them. The truth is that children are tuned into what is happening. The best way to normalize the situation is by communication.

Many professionals believe that communication with children is best done by parents or relatives. However, family members point out that the ability of relatives to explain brain injury depends on their understanding of it and on their emotional condition. Relatives under stress often do not retain explanations of medical terms and procedures. Others can repeat what has been reported, but do not grasp its meaning. Consequently, many family members are the last to get accurate medical information. While young children may be less interested in the medical details, they still worry about, "What will Daddy or Mommy be like?"

Protecting children by not talking with them can lead to more confusion and increase fears. Well meaning platitudes such as, "Everything will be all right" may not be reassuring to a child who can see the worry and distress among relatives and friends. This platitude may also turn out to be untrue.

Age Matters

All communication with children must fit their level of language, comprehension and maturation. Young children need very concrete explanations. All children need repeated opportunities to receive information, ask questions, express fears, and have time to absorb what has happened.

Age makes a difference. It is a factor in deciding if and when to allow or encourage a child to visit a parent in the hospital or rehabilitation program. Families need to consider how a parent's condition and appearance may affect a child.

Putting added pressure on children during a parent's absence by saying, "You are the man of the house while Daddy is in the hospital" or "Mommy needs you to be the lady of the house now" can be disastrous. The child may be overwhelmed by thoughts like, "Will my family survive?" Expecting your child to be brave or assume even more responsibility is unfair.

Helping the younger child

Young children do not intellectually process sorrow and may not understand their feelings. They do not have a basis to compare what they feel with what is normal.

Children may display more, not fewer, signs of mourning six months after a loss occurs. It is common for a child to regress when grieving. A younger child may become overdependent, demand constant attention and want others to do things that they are capable of (like tying shoelaces). A child's grief may result in explosive emotions of anger or feelings of hate, blame, rage and jealousy. These feelings can be directed toward the non-injured parent, a teacher, playmates or the world in general.

Some children do not keep their grief front and center, but pace themselves. Just because they are able to play or watch their favorite television show does not mean that they are not upset. Their world is primarily a world of play and that is where they retreat.

Young children may find it hard to know what is going on as they are shuttled between temporary caregivers and relatives. Even the youngest child can benefit from being involved by drawing get well cards, making cassette tapes and telephone calls. Not visiting can be isolating, but the first visit with a parent after a brain injury can be confusing and frightening if the child is not prepared and supported.

Helping the youth or adolescent

Teenagers may be embarrassed by their injured parent's behavior and they may feel angry at how life has changed. Feelings of guilt or frustration may build or emerge over time. They may not understand why it's bothering them years later. They may "hate" the life they have. New financial strains from medical expenses and lost income may mean adolescents can't keep up with peers and may result in feeling left out. Let them know that how they feel is perfectly normal.

When a parent has an illness, coming home usually means returning to routines. Coming home after a brain injury is different as the parent may not be able to resume routine activities. Changes in a parent's behavior, communication, social skills, physical abilities or thinking may influence a teenager's willingness to have friends visit or go out with the parent. Prepare adolescents to anticipate and respond to comments, questions or jokes about how their parent looks, behaves, moves, speaks and thinks.

Rehabilitation can take months and/or years. It's important for the non-injured parent and children to find ways to care for themselves. This may be through exercise, mini-vacations, hobbies or entertainment. Assure family members there is no need to feel guilty about having a good time. They deserve to live their lives as fully as possible.

Helping the young adult

Young adults who were planning or expecting to leave home prior to a parent's injury may have mixed feelings about leaving now. Some choose to leave, others stay. Adult children already living away from home when a parent is injured may emotionally distance themselves while others find ways to be involved. Some juggle competing demands between the needs of their own families and their parents.

Hospital and Rehabilitation

Tips for families on helping children visit...

✓ Explain what a coma is.

✓ Ask for written information for children on brain injury.

✓ Explain how the room and equipment look, sound, and smell.

✓ Describe how a parent will look, behave and react.

✓ Show how to comfort a parent by simple actions such as touching, holding hands, talking or reading.

✓ Don't force visiting – let the child choose if and when.

Tips for families on helping children cope...

✓ Be flexible. Do not assume that children can or want to keep up with normal schedules. Keeping them busy in a routine to avoid their feelings is problematic. Children react to acute stress. They may have difficulty concentrating, getting organized or absorbing information.

✓ Allow children to ask questions and ensure them that no question is "too silly" or "none of their business."

✓ Enlist the help of friends and relatives who can take children to prescheduled events, if they want to go.

✓ Ask friends to relieve the non-injured parent at the hospital so the parent can go home or attend activities with children.

✓ Find ways for children to still have fun.

Tips for health care professionals at the hospital...

✓ Ask what family members have been told.

✓ Help explain terms, procedures and tests.

✓ Meet with the uninjured parent and children to explain what has happened and what will happen next.

✓ Give family members time and opportunities to ask questions.

✓ Use terms and language that can be understood and is appropriate for their age.

✓ Show pictures and diagrams with written information.

✓ Explain what their parent is doing when they ask, i.e. let them walk in the parallel bars, ride in a wheelchair, etc.

✓ Keep information simple when the family's stress is high. Give more details to children when they are prepared and ready to hear and learn more.

✓ Provide materials written specifically for families and children.

✓ Explain how a parent may act and what help will be needed at home.

✓ Don't be afraid to say, "I don't know."

Back Home and in the Community

A parent's return home from the hospital or rehabilitation marks the beginning of the next stage of recovery. This means changes for everyone.

Tips for families when the parent comes home...

✓ Be prepared to make major adjustments.

✓ Communicate and encourage children to disclose fears, wishes and dreams.

✓ Consider counseling to help a child cope and grieve.

✓ Allow and encourage safe and appropriate ways for children to express their feelings.

✓ Don't let children get lost in the shuffle; save some time every day for each child.

✓ Let friends and family help ease the burden.

Tips for families on talking with friends and peers...

✓ Offer to meet with friends, peers and/or teachers to explain what has happened and its effects on the family.

✓ Encourage questions and answer as honestly as you can.

✓ Activate a support system for your children (i.e. ask friends, a favorite teacher, the parent of a close friend to spend time with your child and be a sounding board).

Tips for professionals on getting help for families...

✓ Explain benefits of receiving help from a professional, especially one who understands brain injury.

✓ Emphasize that obtaining outside help is not a sign of weakness but rather of sign of caring and looking after one's self.

✓ Ask the Brain Injury Association in your state or province about resources or programs for family members.

Helping the Child at School

School can be a welcome escape from the stress of hospital visits and disruptions at home. This may be the one area in a child's life that does not change. However, school can be a source of additional stress if teachers are unaware of the student's needs for support and guidance.

Tips for school staff...

✓ Ask how the student is - the family's emotional trauma is just as real as the physical injuries.
✓ Reach out to the student whose parent has been injured.
✓ Gather information on brain injury to educate school staff.
✓ Be alert for changes in grades and behavior and communicate concerns with the family.
✓ Watch for signs of depression and grief.
✓ Consider counseling and guidance services to support the student.

Conclusion

Many family members speak of the appreciation they gained for the fragility of life and their gratitude that their parent survived. They have an increased awareness of what it means to live with a disability and the need for compassion and understanding.

Resources

Military One Source - serving American troops and families

www.militaryonesource.com 800-342-9647

The Military Injured Joint Support operations center (24/7 family support)

Veterans Affairs

Describes services for veterans and has a page for children. www.va.gov and www.va.gov/kids

References

Breese Biagioni, J. (2004). *A Change of Mind: One family's journey through brain injury.* Wake Forest, NC: Lash and Associates Publishing/Training, Inc.

Lash, M. (1993). *When a Parent Has a Brain Injury: Sons and daughters speak out.* Worcester, MA: Brain Injury Association of Massachusetts.

Loss, Grief & Mourning
After Brain Injury
Written by: Janelle Breese Biagioni

✓ experience of grief
✓ primary and secondary losses
✓ possible responses of grief
✓ importance of grieving and mourning

Physical Death vs. Non-physical Death

Death is most commonly associated with loss. Physical death brings great losses to family and friends. Non-physical deaths or endings can also bring loss. Their impact may not be as obvious to others. Yet it is still painful for those going through a life-altering ordeal.

It is important to grieve and mourn because that is how people heal and move forward in life. A person can feel loss through many different events including:

- death
- divorce
- separation
- illness
- injury
- transitions (i.e. loss of employment, empty-nest syndrome, geographical moves)

There is a connection between brain injury and grief and it is important for individuals and families to do the work of healing.

Bereavement, Grieving, and Mourning

They are not the same. These words are used interchangeably; however, they have different meanings. Dr. Alan Wolfelt, of the Center for Loss and Life Transition in Fort Collins, CO, defines bereavement, grieving, and mourning as follows.

Bereavement is the *call.*

It is the event that causes a loss (death, injury, ending of a relationship, etc.).

Grieving is the *internal response* to loss.

It is how one feels on the inside (sad, angry, confused, afraid, alone, etc.).

Mourning is the *external response* to the loss.

It is how one expresses feelings about the loss (funerals, ceremonies, rituals, talking, writing, etc.).

Primary and Secondary Losses

People who have a brain injury, their family and friends, and even their co-workers, may find themselves grappling with grief because of the primary and secondary losses that can follow a brain injury. The impact that a brain injury has on an individual's life can be staggering. The day-to-day challenges and life-altering changes for a survivor of brain injury can be overwhelming. The catastrophic injury results in the *primary loss.*

Secondary losses come after the primary loss. They can be physical, emotional, spiritual, financial, and social losses. These are the *secondary losses.*

The person with the brain injury, as well as every person in the family, will start on a journey of grief and mourning. It is important to acknowledge and encourage this. But this journey is not restricted to the individual and family. Others who are involved with the person (co-workers, friends, and extended family) may also grieve and mourn.

Everyone who is connected to the person with a brain injury may be affected in some way. For example, a spouse may have to quit a job to become a caregiver. Loss of employment and income are secondary losses for the spouse and family. It is also the loss of the relationship between husband and wife that existed prior to the injury. A spouse may have to give up outside activities. These are losses of social and community connections. Not only should each person explore any losses, but each person must find appropriate and safe ways to express their feelings of grief.

Ability to grieve

The ability to grieve has little to do with a person's capacity to understand. Rather, it has to do with the ability to feel. If a person has the ability to love, then the person has the ability to feel sorrow and the need to grieve and mourn a loss. This is especially true for children. They may not understand what is happening. They may not be able to verbalize their feelings. But they have the ability to feel, and therefore, they need to grieve and mourn too. An injury to a sibling or parent is a life altering event for a child.

The Grief Journey

The journey through grief is a *process* – not an event. Grieving and mourning take time. Grief is often ongoing for months and sometimes, years. Grieving a loss is not done in a step-by-step fashion. The grief journey is unpredictable. On some days, individuals may find themselves feeling stronger, happier, and accepting. Then they find themselves in a state of disbelief, confusion, and sadness on the next day. The grief journey can feel like a person is walking in a fog. The *familiar* is no longer *familiar*. Everyone does not grieve in the same way. Many factors can influence how a person grieves and mourns, such as family history, faith or religious upbringing, and support systems.

Responses to grief

Individuals can have a wide-range of responses to grief including:

- shock
- numbness
- disbelief
- disorganization
- confusion
- searching for meaning
- anxiety
- guilt
- regret
- panic and
- fear

Grief may bring about physical changes, explosive emotions, and feelings of emptiness and sadness. The ultimate goal of the grief journey is *NOT* to "get over" the pain and loss. Rather, the goal is to reconcile, heal and integrate the loss into one's life so that a person can once again embrace joy. Grieving families need the opportunity to say, "Hello – Goodbye – Hello." This means saying goodbye to the life they once had so they can embrace the life they have now.

Feelings of R.A.G.E.

Survivors of brain injury and their families are often caught off-guard by their response to loss. Having a sense of *"I'm going crazy"* or *"I'm not doing this right!"* are common. Other universal feelings are:

R – Regret – *"Why did I let him drive?" "I never said good-bye."*

A – Anger – *"Why did this happen to us?" "How could she have been so careless?"*

G – Guilt – *"I should have stopped him." "I shouldn't get so frustrated with her."*

E – Emotions – *"I feel so sad." "I feel lost." "I am afraid."*

Types of Mourning

Mourning is the expression of one's feelings of grief. It can be done through rituals, ceremonies, writing, and talking to name a few ways. There are circumstances when expressing these feelings can be difficult and may even be prohibited.

Complicated Mourning is more severe than grief. It is different from depression. It is when the usual or common feelings of disbelief, loss, and anguish do not fade or soften over time. It is when these feelings persist for years. Similar to a chronic distressed state, it creates a new and more despondent frame of mind.

People in this state need lasting support and professional advice. If left unaddressed, complicated grief and mourning can lead to depression, suicide, drug and alcohol abuse and other health issues (i.e. heart disease). Researchers at the University of Pittsburgh found that 51% of patients treated with a therapy developed specifically for the symptoms of complicated grief showed improvement.

Extraordinary Mourning is not the same as complicated mourning. Extraordinary mourning essentially means *unusual emotional distress caused by bereavement.* Grief after brain injury often falls into this category. It is challenging for families to address the "non-physical" death that can arise from brain injury. Because they often *look* like the same family as before, society holds a false expectation that they _should/can_ function as the same family. The secondary losses experienced by each person in the family also require exploration and expression.

Doing the Work

Grieving and mourning are hard work. The only way to the other side is through it. You cannot go over, under, or sidestep grief. You must go through it to get beyond it. If you choose to avoid the work of healing, you face potential pitfalls such as substance abuse, destructive relationships, and health issues. By choosing to do the work of grieving, you are giving yourself permission to live.

Tips for persons with brain injury to grieve and mourn losses...

✓ Be gentle with yourself – grieving can be physically, spiritually, and emotionally draining.
✓ Do not diminish how you feel about what has happened and don't allow others to underrate your loss either. Your loss is real.
✓ Take time to work through your feelings about what has happened and how it affects you.
✓ Recognize that you may have secondary losses (i.e. loss of income, loss of friends, and loss of lifestyle).
✓ Recognize that your family is also experiencing grief. They need time to work through their emotions and may do it differently than you do.
✓ Find appropriate and safe ways to express your grief. It is essential to your well-being.
✓ Take time to reflect on who you were before your injury, who you are now, and who you want to be in the future.
✓ Ask for help – you do not need to do this alone.
✓ Keep life in perspective so that grieving and mourning do not totally overwhelm you.

Tips for family members to grieve and mourn their losses...

✓ Recognize your personal losses which may include loss of an equal partner in your relationship, loss of income and lifestyle, and loss of the family as you once knew it. Understand that you have the right to grieve and mourn your losses.
✓ Find someone to share your grief with (i.e. family, friend, professional, support group).
✓ Have courage. Your life, as is life for your loved one, is different. That realization can be painful.

✓ Allow yourself to seek respite or relief. You need time to feel what you are feeling and to express those feelings.
✓ Ask for help – you do not need to do this alone.
✓ Keep life in perspective so that grieving and mourning do not totally overwhelm you.

Tips for professionals to support survivors and families in the grief process... S.H.A.R.E.

S – Support (engage in short and long-term supports)

Ensure that grieving survivors and family members have short-term and long-term supports. Often family and friends rally around them immediately following the injury, but they may fade away over time. They may no longer be available for support as life calls them back to _their own_ commitments. Survivors of brain injury and their families need ongoing support throughout rehabilitation and recovery. Support can come from individuals, groups, and professionals.

H – Hope (thread or sense that some good will return in your life)

People need to be reassured that they will have help along the way. They need reassurance that while this is painful today, working through their grief will eventually lead to acceptance of the changes in their lives.

A – Acknowledge (life before the event, life at present, life in the future)

Encourage survivors and families to talk about what their life was like before the injury, what life is like now, and what they want in the future. This can bring a wide range of feelings to the surface. It is important to help people find safe and appropriate ways to express those feelings (i.e. journaling, talking, art).

R – Reflection (spiritual, memories, planning)

Personal reflection is an important part of the grief journey. It can be a painful examination. However, searching for meaning and understanding of what has happened in one's life is a critical part of the grief journey.

E – Engage in Life (reconnect to loved ones, friends, co-workers, and community)

Survivors and their families often feel disconnected to one another. Their extended family and friends may not understand what they are going through. They cannot be expected to "carry on" as they had before the injury. It is only after they are allowed to work through their grief that they can come to a place of acceptance and then begin engaging in life again.

Conclusion

Individuals with brain injury and their families may experience loss on many levels, including physical, social, spiritual, and emotional changes. It is essential that they be allowed to recognize their losses and express the feelings connected with each loss.

References

Breese Biagioni, J. (2004). *A Change of Mind: One Family's Journey through Brain Injury.* Wake Forest, NC: Lash and Associates Publishing/Training Inc.

Wolfelt, A. (1992). *Understanding Grief: Helping Yourself Heal.* Florence, KY: Accelerated Development.

Depression

After Brain Injury
Written by: Pamela Law, Ph.D.

✓ recognize symptoms of depression
✓ know when and how to ask for help
✓ locate helpful resources

Signs of Depression

Brain injury is so sudden and unpredictable that it is a truly devastating experience for many individuals and their families. People often feel as if the rug has been ripped out from beneath them and they do not know how or when they will get their footing back.

It is not unusual for the individual who has been injured, or for family members, to feel depressed after such a traumatic experience.

Facts about depression and brain injury

- People with brain injury are more likely to feel depressed than people without brain injury.
- Some people feel depressed and anxious at the same time.
- These feelings may occur right after the injury or they can surface months or even years later.
- Some forms of depression only last for a short time, while other forms may last for a long time.
- People who are aware of the losses and changes in their lives may be more likely to show signs of depression after a brain injury.

Everybody gets the blues now and then. This is normal. Depression is different. It is a more extensive reaction. The person has a low or depressed mood. There may be a marked lack of interest or pleasure in activities that the person normally enjoys. It is a sign of depression when these feelings are present most of the day, nearly every day, for at least two weeks.

A person who is depressed may also show changes in at least four of the following patterns of behavior.

Check the boxes that apply to you or your family member.

☐ Major change in appetite (eating more or eating less)
☐ Big weight loss not caused by deliberate dieting or a big weight gain
☐ Lack of sleep or excessive sleep
☐ Moving slower or faster than usual
☐ Loss of energy, feeling fatigued
☐ Feelings of worthlessness or excessive guilt
☐ Difficulty making decisions or reduced concentration

Depression can result in a person...

☐ Becoming angry or upset, crying, or feeling numb

☐ Having trouble managing these feelings and controlling when they occur

☐ Having nightmares or difficulty sleeping

☐ Feeling tired all the time even after enough sleep

☐ Feeling that life has lost its purpose

☐ Being unable to appreciate the good things in life

☐ Enjoying being with others less and avoiding social situations

☐ Getting into frequent conflicts with friends and family members

☐ Finding it difficult to get going in the morning or to complete tasks

☐ Trying to "self-medicate" by turning to drugs or alcohol

☐ Engaging in thrill seeking behaviors, such as spending too much, taking chances such as driving fast, or dramatically increasing sexual activity

☐ Reporting medical symptoms that feel real but have no physical basis

☐ Hurting oneself

☐ Having persistent thoughts of self-destruction which need to be closely watched

How to Help

There are many things you can do to help relieve symptoms of depression, as well as things to avoid.

Tips for what to DO...

✓ Take care of your needs now.

   This includes eating and drinking wisely, making time for solitude, and keeping a normal routine.

✓ Understand that you will feel a wide range of feelings, including anger.

   Give yourself time to experience and understand these feelings.

✓ Seek help.

   Find a trusted friend, family member, support group, counselor or therapist who can help you express your emotions of sadness, anger, frustration or disappointment. Feeling that you are all alone and with no one to turn to will probably make your pain worse.

✓ Find a support group.

   Others who have gone through the emotional and physical trauma of a brain injury can share valuable experience and perspectives. Call the Brain Injury Association in your state to locate a support group for individuals or families.

✓ Post numbers of friends, family, doctor, and pastor near your telephone.

✓ Ask for a hug. Every hug dilutes pain.

✓ Tell your story.

   This is part of your healing journey. It is your way of making sense out of what has happened to you. It can help you put events in order. Your story will likely change over time, not necessarily about what happened, but in what you choose to focus on now. Telling your story helps you figure out what you are struggling with today. Not telling your story depletes your energy.

✓ Remember that, even when it seems you have no choice, you always have a choice.

   Choose healing by nurturing your own needs. Find out what makes your spirit soar and let yourself do those things. Cry if you need to. Laugh if you want to.

✓ Search for answers to your deepest and burning questions.

   There are no stupid questions. If a question is nagging at you, then it is worth asking. Some questions may be unanswerable. Life is indeed a mystery and it is more fully lived by journeying into that mystery.

✓ Say out loud, "I will get through this!"

Tips for what to avoid or WHAT NOT TO DO...

✓ Stay away from friends.

✓ Use drugs, alcohol or other short-term relieving behaviors like sex, spending money or work to hide your feelings.

✓ Be afraid to ask for help.

✓ Think your feelings are a sign of weakness.

✓ Drive. Driving and grief do not mix well. Take advantage of offers for transportation.

✓ Refuse help.

✓ Don't hurt yourself. If you feel an impulse to hurt yourself, call a loved one or 911.

When Should I Seek Treatment?

While comfort from friends and family members can help, there are times when professional treatment is needed. This applies to the individual with a brain injury and to family members. This is especially true if any of you are continuing to have some of the difficulties already described and if they are interfering with your ability to meet the challenges and demands of daily life. It is important to seek treatment if you find yourself engaging in, or often thinking about, self-destructive behavior such as reliance on drugs, alcohol, thrill seeking, or harming yourself.

Seeking help can be difficult. Some people think that seeking professional treatment is a sign of weakness. Some find it makes them feel very vulnerable. A professional who has experience treating people with brain injury will understand how and why your life has changed. The professional may be a psychologist, social worker, therapist, rehabilitation counselor or psychiatrist. Regardless of the profession, the skilled counselor who understands brain injury can help you and your family better understand your feelings and offer helpful strategies and support.

Sometimes medication can help. Your counselor or therapist can work with your physician or psychiatrist to determine if medication is needed to treat your depressed mood and to help you function and participate in life more fully. When properly prescribed, medication is not a crutch. It can be a valuable tool that can raise your mood and energy to help you function more effectively throughout the day. It can also help you participate in counseling.

Counseling can feel hard and even painful at times. Talking about your losses and pain can renew feelings of sadness. Your counselor or therapist can help you express your feelings in a safe and supportive environment. Your tears will be welcomed. Sometimes people feel like they are getting worse at first as they begin to talk about and share the feelings that are part of the depression. It is important to "stick with it" in counseling. The only way out of depression is to go straight through your feelings of sadness.

For many of us, we are our own worst critic. We say things to ourselves that we would never say to someone we love. If this is true for you, your counselor will work with you to replace negative and self-defeating self-talk with realistic self-talk and appraisals. This can improve your ability to cope with stress. You will also learn new ways to cope with depression and practice them in your everyday life.

Families are very important. Just as the person who has had a brain injury is struggling to put life back together, family members are doing the same. There are many counseling options that family members can choose. They may decide to see a counselor separately or they may elect to have joint counseling with the relative who has been injured. They may choose to do both. Couples and/or family sessions can build upon individual sessions. This is an opportunity to learn conflict resolution skills, to communicate better, to compromise, and to be assertive without being aggressive. Couples and family sessions can offer everyone the opportunity to speak freely without fear. It is an opportunity to strengthen relationships even during this stressful and difficult period.

Summary

Depression after brain injury is, unfortunately, remarkably common among individuals and family members. It is frequently the result of the depressing circumstances you may have found yourself in after a brain injury. Depression does not mean you are "crazy." Rather, it is a natural reaction to an overwhelming and unexpected situation.

Seeking professional help is not a sign of weakness or failure. The bravest people are the ones who ask for help when they need it. We are not meant to go through the devastation of depression and brain injury alone. Know that it is a sign of strength and courage to seek help in managing your symptoms of depression. It is important not to go it alone, especially when you have thoughts of hurting yourself or a loved one. There are many services and supports available to you and your family to help manage depression after brain injury. When in doubt, reach out and ask for help.

Take an active role in your care and work with others. There are many resources available within your community. These include local brain injury associations, hospitals and programs serving people who experience disability following brain injury. There are emergency crisis centers, self-help groups, community mental health centers, telephone information lines, and crisis hot lines. The list below is a place to start.

National Resources

Brain Injury Association of USA
1-800-444-6443   www.biausa.org

National Depressive & Manic Depressive Assoc.
1-800-82-NDMDA   www.ndmda.org

National Foundation for Depressive Illness
1-800-248-4344   www.depression.org

National Institute of Mental Health
1-800-647-2642   www.nimh.nih.gov

National Mental Health Association
1-800-969-6642   www.nmha.org

National Resource Center on Homelessness and
    Mental Illness
1-800-444-7415   ww.nrchmi.samhsa.gov

Panic Disorder Information Line
1-800-64-PANIC   www.panic.thetazzone.com

Suicide Prevention Advocacy Network
1-888-649-1366   www.spanusa.org

References

Jongsma, A.E. & Peterson, M. (1999). *The Complete Adult Psychotherapy Treatment Planner Second Edition.* NY: John Wiley & Sons.

Kubler-Ross, E. & Kessler, D. (2005). *On Grief and Grieving.*NY: Simon & Schuster.

Walton, C. (1996). When *There Are No Words.* Ventura, CA: Pathfinder.

Worden, J.W. (2002*). Grief Counseling and Grief Therapy Third Edition.* New York: Springer Publishing.

Yalom, I.D. (2002). *The Gift of Therapy: An Open Letter to a New Generation of Therapists and Their Patients.* NY: Harper Collins.

Emotions
Hope after Brain Injury
Written by: Ann V. Deaton, Ph.D.

✓ hold on to hope and emotions
✓ focus on future possibilities
✓ recognize and value what is good

Emotional Reactions

When an individual has a brain injury, most families go through the entire range of emotions. There is fear, anger, hope, despair, and even joy at times. These emotions are often seen as negative (fear, despair, anger) or positive (joy and hope). Each emotion affects how a family member acts and responds to others. This tip card will help you use your emotions effectively rather than allowing them to control or overwhelm you.

You may have felt like you were on a roller coaster of emotions soon after the brain injury occurred. Every day there were unfamiliar terms, complicated medical information and difficult questions that often could not be answered. Your emotions may change over time but they continue to be powerful feelings. Every member of your family may feel a wide range of emotions. Some may be similar to yours; others may be different. All emotions need to be respected. It's important to let everyone in your family know that it's okay to feel angry, afraid, sad, helpless, and overwhelmed. *It's what you do with these emotions that matters.*

Negative Emotions

Anger, sadness, and fear can be negative and destructive. But without them, you would lose valuable energy and perspective. They can help you not only survive, but thrive in the aftermath of a brain injury to a member of your family.

Anger

Most of us try to avoid feeling angry because it's upsetting. We think of anger as aggression, attacking or fighting. It can drive others away. But anger is also a source of incredible energy.

Feeling angry is a common reaction after brain injury. Family members may become angry when an injury was caused by the negligence of others, or by a family member's high risk behavior. In the early days of hospital care, families are often angered when physicians are not readily available or when visiting hours limit time with the injured person. Anger can resurface when progress in rehabilitation falls short of hopes and expectations.

This anger is a natural result of the situation. Its energy can be channeled and used. Anger can lead to determined action and fighting for your rights. It provides an incentive to advocate for what is needed. What could be more valuable with the many challenges you may face after brain injury?

Sadness

Any family member may feel overwhelmed by sadness. It can shut a person down emotionally and physically. Many people feel vulnerable when sad and withdraw, even when they are most in need of support from others.

Sadness is a normal reaction to brain injury and the loss you've experienced. You need support, information, and time to understand and cope with the changes. You may want the help and support of others to get through this painful time. Or you may want to be left alone when sad. People often become more willing to ask for help to get through this difficult time – whether it is from a spouse, close friend, clergy, or counselor.

Fear

This is a natural early reaction to learning of a family member's brain injury. Fear is our expectation of pain and loss. The situation often appears much worse when a person is fearful.

All families have some fear of the unknown after brain injury. It is particularly difficult when professionals treating the person are unable to tell the family what the future holds. Expecting the worst-case scenario can make a family feel even more fearful.

This fear can push you to seek answers and give you the energy to ask questions, find information and make contacts. Seeking knowledge is empowering. It can be the key to overcoming fear. Recognizing your fears can also help you identify risks and avoid dangerous situations.

Positive Emotions

More comfortable for us are the emotions we think of as positive. These emotions can help you over the course of brain injury recovery. Joy and love are two examples.

Joy

This feels like openness, relaxation, and happiness. It offers a break and escape from sadness and worry. It is a welcome opportunity to feel glad to be alive and full of energy. Families may feel great joy as the individual with a brain injury reaches milestones in recovery and learns to walk, talk, or work again. There are, however, limits of joy. It usually comes and goes over the course of brain injury recovery.

Love

Loving a person with a brain injury can help that person gain confidence and the willingness to get through the difficult and challenging parts of recovery. Love means accepting and treasuring another person. Loving without conditions is an incredible support to the person who has been injured. Again, love has limits. Unconditional love supports the person with a brain injury. But love alone is not always enough to urge the person to take on difficult challenges or to overcome the odds.

All emotions, whether we see them as positive or negative, are responses to life experiences. You may feel all these emotions as you and your family try to cope with what it means to have a brain injury.

Using Emotion Instead of Letting It Control You

Using your emotions first requires that you be aware of them. Only then can you choose how to use them. Awareness is gained by questioning your experience, by focusing on it and trying to identify what your emotions are and what triggers them.

Are you afraid? What is it that you fear? Are you afraid of building the ramp to your house because it may mean your family member will never walk again? Build it anyway. Use your fear to get answers, to fully explore the situation and minimize the risks. Even though you may still feel afraid, you may decide that it is worth taking the risk.

Tips for handling your emotions…

✓ Stay in the moment.

Rather than wishing for the moment to pass, ask yourself what exactly this moment is about.

✓ Allow emotions to subside or quiet.

Instead of trying to hold onto an emotion, be aware when it lessens. Notice the emotion that replaces it. Why this emotion now? What triggered it? How can it help you?

✓ Review and reflect.

Keep a journal of your different emotions and experiences. It is often easier to understand your feelings after some time has passed. Reading your journal days, weeks, months or even years later gives you a different outlook. This can help you understand what you were feeling and why. Review and reflection can help you use your emotions effectively or change them.

✓ Find someone you trust.

If you are feeling overwhelmed by an emotion, share it with someone you trust. Ask for the person's views and ideas. By sharing the emotion, you will find it more manageable and less overwhelming.

✓ Consider the opposite emotion.

Sometimes an emotion can block you from taking action. Or it may be prevent you from getting action from someone else. When this happens, try choosing the opposite emotion and ask yourself what you'd do if you felt that way instead. For example, if you are feeling angry but need to make a request, ask yourself, "How would I say this if I were feeling warmly towards this person?"

Focusing Your Emotions

All emotions have value, but forgiveness, hope, and gratitude are important for helping you and your family recover from a brain injury and cope with its effects.

Forgiveness

Holding onto blame and resentment can damage your body, your relationships, and your ability to move ahead. Yet forgiveness often seems impossible when an injury was avoidable or preventable. Letting go and forgiving are essential to your emotional recovery and to helping the person who has survived.

Tips for families on forgiveness...

"It was hard for me to forgive my husband, because I didn't want him to join the reserves. I was afraid he would be called up for the war and I was pregnant. We argued about it a lot."

What does it take to forgive? While the process may be different for each person, here are some options...

✓ Recognize the amount of effort you are putting into maintaining resentment. What would it be like if you had that energy available for something else?

✓ Realize that by continuing to focus on who's at fault, you are unable to accept the changes in the person who has been injured. How would that person feel to be fully accepted, valued, and loved?

Find forgiveness for:

- yourself
- other family members
- the person with a brain injury
- the circumstances of the injury
- those who don't understand.

Forgiveness opens up more positive possibilities for the future and maximizes available energy.

Hope

"For a while, hope was all we had to hold on to and it got us through the darkest days. Without hope, I couldn't have gone on."

Hope is a belief that a situation will improve. It is a state of optimism, of looking ahead and seeing that good things can happen. Many people see hope as the opposite of despair. Hope offers possibility and provides a vision for a future. There is positive energy with hope that encourages a person to persist in reaching for a goal.

Tips for families on hope...

✓ Evaluate information as you receive it and be realistic.

The potential for brain injury recovery is often underestimated by those with limited experience of long term recovery.

✓ The seeds of the future are here in the present.

Recognize what's good already. Notice the person's strengths and resilience.

✓ Recognize that small miracles happen each day.

"I hope for a full recovery but, to be honest, he's already done far more than I imagined. I just hope for his happiness as life goes on."

Gratitude

"I was so grateful that my wife was alive. That meant everything to me."

Gratitude comes with appreciating the present moment. It is being thankful for *what is* rather than wishing for what is not. Gratitude is a state of being in which a feeling of peace is possible. Gratitude does not mean there are no challenges ahead. It may, in fact, mean that you find yourself able to accept the challenges and to live in each moment as you experience what life has to offer.

"Life is not the same for any of us, but I am still grateful for each improvement I see in my son, no matter how big or small. I don't take anything for granted now."

Conclusion

Your emotions will be your changing but constant companion through your family's recovery from brain injury. Hold onto your hope and optimism and use them to fuel your continuous movement forward. Recognize negative emotions and harness the energy they provide to take action and accomplish incredible things. Always recognize and value what is good in your life today, as well as the possibilities for what's ahead of you.

References

Emerald, D. (2006). *The Power of TED* (*The Empowerment Dynamic*). Bainbridge Island, WA: Polaris Publishing.

Groopman, J. (2005). *The Anatomy of Hope.* New York: Random House, Inc.

Zander, R.S. & Zander, B. (2000). *The Art of Possibility.* Boston: Harvard Business School Press.

Caregiving After Brain Injury
A Survival Guide
Written by: Carolyn Rocchio, Parent

✓ gives caregiving techniques
✓ describes cognitive needs
✓ identifies helpful resources
✓ cares for the caretaker

Caregiving by Families

Caregiving is a very special service that can take many forms for families after a member has a brain injury. It can feel rewarding, frustrating, confusing, overwhelming, satisfying, exhausting - and meaningful. Caregiving is very hard work.

The period of recovery and rehabilitation following a brain injury varies. Some individuals may need only a short period of nurturing and physical assistance to reenter the mainstream of life. Others with more severe injuries may require more assistance. Some will need help for the rest of their lives. Others will need physical help, supervision for safety, or help communicating. Some will need help with judgment, reasoning, and organizational skills. Because each brain injury is different, each person needs different assistance and support from a caregiver.

A new type of caregiving

Mothers are the stereotypical caregivers used to nurturing family members through illnesses or after surgery. Famous American artist, Norman Rockwell, painted the mother/caregiver carrying hot soup to a sick child's bedside. The bed was strewn with books and games to entertain the ailing child and there were bottles of medication on the table for a quick recovery.

Caregiving for a person with a brain injury is very different from that image. Most persons with a brain injury are not in bed for a long time. They may not even be sick or physically impaired. Their appearance of physical recovery or well-being often makes it harder for others to recognize their needs for assistance and support.

Caregivers find that changes in how an individual thinks and learns after a brain injury can make it more difficult for the person to initiate, organize, and follow through with what were previously very simple tasks such as:

- bathing and personal care
- dressing for weather conditions
- structuring and planning daily activities
- meal planning and preparation
- time management
- proper use of medication
- transportation
- recreation and socialization
- money management
- use of leisure time

From rehabilitation to home

Knowing how much assistance to volunteer without assuming too much responsibility can be a difficult balancing act for the caregiver. If you have been involved in the rehabilitation process, you may be familiar with what your family member can do safely and independently and when help is needed. Giving physical help or care may be just the beginning. You can make your job easier by gathering information about your family member's cognitive abilities and difficulties. Ask the professionals involved about how these changes affect your family member's thinking, behavior and vision.

Rehabilitation programs usually give individuals with brain injury a highly structured environment. It is important to keep this consistency at home. As a person is discharged, information about medications and follow up appointments is usually given. It is important that families/caregivers also be instructed about:

- use, care and maintenance of special appliances, i.e., wheelchairs, walkers, braces and crutches
- amount of structure and monitoring required for safety
- cognitive strategies for all members of the household

- behavioral management techniques to ensure consistent reinforcement
- choosing one person in the family to be the "case manager" or authority figure.

Changes at Home and in the Community

Caregiving responsibilities change over time as the individual with a brain injury changes. Many caregivers find that they have to reevaluate periodically what the person needs because the situation has changed.

Signs of change that professional help is needed are...

- changes in behavior, particularly if the situation is becoming harder to control
- increased confusion, loss of balance or disorientation, particularly if your family member has a shunt
- refusal to take prescribed medications
- leaving home without permission or a reason
- changes in sleep habits, either insomnia or sleeping too much
- use of street drugs or alcohol.

It is wise to seek help in managing these changes. This helps everyone living in the home and can prevent the situation from getting out of control.

Caregiving demands a great deal emotionally and physically. You may be feeling:

- overwhelmed with so many demands on your time
- guilty that you have no, or little, control over the situation
- helpless and at times hopeless
- embarrassed by some of your family member's actions
- pulled in several directions while trying to meet the needs of everyone in the family
- unsure how long you can continue with no end in sight
- unable to experience joy or happiness.

Caregivers can be under greater than average stress. Some of this stress comes from a lack of closure for your grief. The person has survived the brain injury but you have lost the person who once was. These feelings, often called "mobile mourning," are normal. They can come and go but often continue over time.

It is vitally important that you take care of yourself. That can be very difficult, particularly when others in the family are working or you are the sole caregiver. Stress can be very damaging to the body, particularly the immune system. A University of California study recently reported that chronic stress appears to accelerate the aging process, shortens the life span of cells and can create an environment that promotes disease. Take steps to find the help you need.

Tips for taking care of yourself...
✓ Make time for yourself, even if it is taking time to read a book for an hour or going to a movie.
✓ Eat properly and take care of yourself even when it is hard to do.
✓ Monitor your health by scheduling routine medical examinations and talk with your doctor.
✓ Include humor in your life, whether it be renting comedies for the family or attending live performances that create a feeling of elation or light-heartedness.

Tips for helping yourself by finding help...
✓ Enlist the support of friends, even a telephone friendship can put you in touch with the outside world.
✓ Give family and friends who want to help suggestions about ways to relieve you.
✓ Take advantage of respite care to the extent it is available in your community.
✓ Share your cares and concerns with others experiencing similar problems by joining a brain injury support group and/or other self-help group.
✓ Seek counseling or help from a trained professional if you experience an emotional meltdown.
✓ Keep a notebook of medication dosages, schedules of activities and names of all treating professionals.
✓ Teach others to do your job should an emergency arise forcing you to find a replacement.

Tips for paying attention to your emotions...
✓ Remain calm when things get out of control; give yourself time to leave the room and regain your composure.
✓ Release your feelings by using a journal - just jotting down a few sentences to describe your day can often help you find something good about life as well as vent the more frustrating events.
✓ Try meditation, yoga or other forms of relaxation.

Sometimes the simplest remedies, when used regularly, can make a difference in how you manage your caregiving. Persons with severe cognitive and behavioral changes often have little control over their lives. Giving them some choices can create a more cooperative spirit. It is usually easier to change the environment than to change the individual.

The following *Seven Things Families Need to Remember* originally appeared on the web site of the Brain Injury Association of America (www.biausa.org). They can help you keep the environment free of hostility and maintain calm.

- ✓ Model behaviors you would like to see.
- ✓ Reinforce behaviors you would like to see increase. Like a garden, "Water the behaviors you'd like to see grow."
- ✓ Structure the environment and use cues for positive behaviors.
- ✓ Plan rest periods.
- ✓ Ignore the behaviors you would like to see decrease when safety is not an issue.
- ✓ Avoid situations that provoke behaviors you are trying to reduce.
- ✓ Redirect the person rather than challenge the person.
- ✓ Seek professional help sooner rather than later.

Caregiving requires a lot of patience and understanding. It is normal to have many feelings that you would prefer to suppress, i.e., resentment, sadness, and grief over the loss of the person you knew and loved before the injury. It is not always easy to learn to love this new and different person. With time, strength and endurance, most caregivers find great comfort in knowing their job is improving the life of their family member with a brain injury.

Caregiver Checklist for Services

It is important to learn about services that can make your job easier and more efficient. Use this list as a guide to check on services that may be available in addition to Veterans' benefits and programs.

- ✓ Was your family member injured before age 22 years? If so, have you contacted your state's Developmental Disabilities Program?
- ✓ If your family member is considering college or vocational training, are you aware of the Rehabilitation Act for and Section 504 for accommodations in academic programs?
- ✓ Do you have or need legal authority, such as guardianship, to manage the business affairs of your family member?

- ✓ Have you applied for state or federal benefits to which your family member may be entitled?
- ✓ If your family member receives financial or disability benefits, do you need a representative payee to help manage funds?
- ✓ Have you explored the availability of state funds to help persons with brain injury?
- ✓ Are there Medicaid waiver programs for brain injury in your state that might provide respite care, companions, or other helpful services?

Caregiver Burnout or Overload

Do not take this lightly. It is time to get professional help if you feel exhausted and are losing interest in life, start your day exhausted or reach a point of despair. Caregivers have more chronic stress in their lives than the general population. It can have a damaging effect on the body. It is important to get to the root cause of the overload, not just look for a quick fix.

Analyzing what you can and cannot control can help pin point the cause of your burn out. Is it your loss of freedom, physical exhaustion, anger about the burden you bear, or other stresses? Try to devise strategies to manage the things you cannot control and find a peaceful compromise with what you are able to control. Faith plays a vital role in quality of life. Spiritual people tend to be optimistic and have more self-esteem and social support. Family caregivers are the unsung heroes of brain injury.

Resources for Caregiver Support

Medical Family Assistance Center (MEDFAC)

866-546-1310

Includes American Red Cross, Legal Assistance Judge Advocate (JAG), financial assistance, community services, etc.

Military One Source - Serving American troops and families

800-342-9647

www.militaryonesource.com

The Military Injured Joint Support Operations Center (24/7 family support).

TRICARE Military Health Services

877-TRICARE (877-874-2273)

www.tricare.osd.mil/hipaa/

www.healthnetfederalservices.com

Veterans Affairs

www.va.gov

National Family Caregivers Association

800-896-3650

www.thefamilycaregiver.org

Respite Resources

You may need respite services or relief care to take some time to renew and energize yourself or in an emergency.

National Respite Locator Service

800-473-1727 ext 222

www.respitelocator.org

Lists respite services, the majority being for children, but includes some providing respite for caregivers of adults and elderly persons.

References

Brain Injury Association of America. Web site: www.biausa.org

Hillocky R. (2000). *Taking Care of Yourself While Providing Care*. Englewood, CO: Craig Hospital.

Matlack J. (2004). *The healing power of prayer. Reader's Digest*. 165(992): 179.

Rocchio C. (2004). *Ketchup on the Baseboard: Rebuilding life after brain injury*. Wake Forest, NC: Lash and Associates Publishing/Training, Inc.

Families as Managers

Of Care and Services
Written by: Marilyn Lash, M.S.W.

✓ helps families communicate effectively
✓ gives tips for negotiating services
✓ shows how to be effective managers

Families as Managers

Few families know what to expect after their spouse, child, sibling or parent survives a brain injury. Many questions arise including...

- What does this mean for our future?
- What kind of help will we need?
- How do I find information?
- Where can I find help?

Professional case managers working in hospitals, rehabilitation programs, insurance companies or agencies can help families with these questions. But over time, the number of experts or professionals involved in the individual's care declines. Yet, families have new questions as they experience the long-term effects of brain injury. Families repeatedly state that they become the managers and coordinators of care and services over time.

This tip card takes the six basic skills used by professional case managers and adapts them for families. They can use these skills to become more effective and efficient managers.

Skill 1: Assessment

How has the brain injury affected my family member?

Professionals have many methods to assess patients or clients. The family's relationship with the person before and after the brain injury is just as important as any formal testing or examination by a clinician. The family still knows this person better than anyone. No one else has your experience and view.

You can start by preparing a brief description of the individual's history, strengths, difficulties and needs. It may take you a while, but getting this down to a 5 minute summary makes it an effective introduction. Practice by developing and rehearsing a short summary that includes:

Information about the injury...
- how long ago it happened
- how the person was hurt
- how serious the injury was
- if the person was in a coma and for how long
- if there were other injuries
- how long the hospital stay was
- if the person was in a rehabilitation program
  (See the tip card *Adults Living with Brain Injury.*)

Describe how the injury has affected...
- academic and career goals
- working and managing money
- living independently
- traveling in the community
- making new friendships and keeping old ones
- having a social life

Practice replying to key questions that professionals ask to learn about a person, including....
- Will you describe the person to me?
- What are his strongest abilities?
- What are her major difficulties?
- What assistance or strategies help him?
- What programs or services is she receiving?
- What else is needed and why?

Tips for describing the effects of the brain injury...
✓ Compare the person before and after the injury.
✓ Identify important changes in the person.
✓ Write down how the person has changed over time.
✓ Describe any changes in behavior and thinking.
✓ Talk to the supervisor if the person is working.
✓ Discuss the injury's effects on employment.
   Ask for copies of medical, rehabilitation and consultant reports and review them.

✓ List confusing terms or jargon and ask professionals to explain them.

✓ Discuss the injury's effects on employment.

Think of assessment as painting a verbal picture or snapshot of the individual. The picture changes depending on who you are talking with and what help is needed. This helps you prepare to seek help from others. Ask yourself, what are the three most important things that I want this person to know? This forces you to prioritize what is most important. The ability to give a clear and accurate description of the person with a brain injury is a valuable skill that you can use repeatedly in meetings, interviews and discussions. Practice doing this with friends and family. Ask for feedback about what's clear and what's confusing.

Skill 2: Information Gathering

What do I need to know?

Figuring out what information you need depends on what you want to accomplish. Getting information is like peeling the layers of an onion. There are federal, state, regional and local programs. There are layers of staff from administrators to direct care staff to clerical workers and volunteers. Funding can be especially complicated. Even learning about eligibility requirements and filing applications can be tedious and involve a lot of paperwork. Here's how you can make sense out of this.

Tips for gathering information...

✓ Describe what you, your family and the person needs.

✓ Learn about programs and services for wounded soldiers and veterans.

✓ List what information to gather and where to get it.

✓ Learn about federal laws affecting persons with disabilities.

✓ Learn about state agencies and programs.

✓ Set up a record keeping system for gathering information.

✓ Identify important contacts with experience and authority for funding.

✓ Copy everything you gather so you can share information with others and not lose the originals.

Ask if the following affect eligibility for services and programs:

- military status
- current age
- age when injured
- type and severity of brain injury and disability
- town or state of residence
- income
- employment
- other sources of income, insurance or benefits.

Keeping track of information can be overwhelming without a system. Take a 3 ring binder and create sections for...

- medical care
- rehabilitation
- veterans and military benefits/programs
- disability/financial benefits
- insurance/medical benefits
- education
- transportation
- advocacy
- recreation
- vocational rehabilitation
- housing
- legal issues

Skill 3: Referral

When do I need to get someone else involved?

A referral to a specialist or program can help, but how do you choose the right one? At the very least, you want someone experienced in brain injury who has worked with other clients or patients of similar age, at similar stages of recovery, and with the particular problem or issue to be addressed.

Tips on questions to ask when considering a referral...

✓ Why is a specialist or program needed?

✓ How is this specialist or program qualified?

✓ When should this referral happen?

✓ What information will the person receiving the referral need?

✓ How is the referral arranged?

✓ What results can I expect?

✓ What will it cost and who pays?

✓ Will there be any follow-up?

✓ What are my alternatives?

Tips to help families make referrals effective...
✓ Identify specific concerns.
✓ Clearly state expected outcomes from the service.
✓ List questions to be answered.
✓ Share information and observations.
✓ Set expectations for communication of findings.
✓ Follow up on recommendations.

Skill 4: Service Coordination

How do I put this all together?

Obtaining more services does not guarantee better care. There is a difference between quality and quantity of services. Coordinating services is critical for reducing stress and maximizing resources. You have many choices. Figure out where and how to focus your time and energy.

Tips on questions to ask about coordinating services...
✓ What services are most important now?
✓ Which services will be most important in the future?
✓ What services are most available?
✓ What services are close by and easy to use?
✓ Which are hardest to find?
✓ What is covered by insurance or other funds?

Skill 5: Advocacy

How do I help others understand what is needed?

"The squeaky wheel gets the grease," is a saying with a lot of truth. But beware of winning the battle but losing the war. Being an effective advocate is more than being assertive and arguing. It requires building relationships, presenting information effectively, knowing your rights, persistence and persuasion. It means learning how you can help people and programs help you!

The most common barriers that families come up against that require advocacy are...
• negative attitudes about people with disabilities and brain injury
• inadequate or inaccurate knowledge about brain injury
• inexperience of staff with cognitive and behavioral effects of brain injury
• lack of money or coverage to pay for services
• an overloaded service delivery system

Tips for being an effective advocate...
✓ Learn about federal laws affecting persons with disabilities.
✓ Gather information from national clearinghouses.
✓ Find other families who are effective advocates and learn from them.
✓ Identify professionals who can support your efforts.
✓ Find out what needs and expectations they have in order to effectively help you.
✓ Talk to others who have used services to find out how effective they are.

Skill 6: Evaluation

Is this working?

Professionals constantly evaluate the progress and abilities of the person with a brain injury. But evaluation is not a job only for clinicians. Families should also evaluate programs and professionals.

Tips on questions for families to ask...
✓ How does this program or service make a difference?
✓ Is the person with a brain injury making progress?
✓ Is this the best program for what the person with a brain injury needs?
✓ Are staff competent?
✓ To what extent does the program/service/professional involve my family?
✓ What are our other options?

Evaluation is not a pass/fail test, but is an opportunity to look at the big picture. Criteria that families have used to evaluate professionals and programs include...
• openness to suggestions
• willingness to try new things
• recognition of person's strengths and accomplishments
• initiative in talking with family
• ability to listen
• consideration of options
• flexibility
• involvement of the person with the brain injury and the family in the whole process.

Conclusion

Families are the constant presence in a sea of changing professionals and services. The challenges of coordinating care and services for a family member with a brain injury can be rewarding and stressful. By using these skills, families can make a difference.

References

Rocchio C, Lash M. (2005) *Life after Brain Injury: A guide for families.* Wake Forest, NC: Lash and Associates Publishing/Training Inc.

COMA
When a Person has a Brain Injury
Written by: Ron Savage, Ed.D. & Marilyn Lash, M.S.W.

✓ understand what coma means
✓ respond and give comfort

What Does Coma Mean?

Being told that your family member, friend or relative is in a coma can be confusing and frightening. Seeing the person unconscious for the first time usually is an emotional shock. The first questions asked are often, "What is a coma? How long will it last? Can he hear me?" Watching and waiting for your relative to respond and become more alert can be emotionally and physically exhausting.

A coma is a state of unresponsiveness that can last for hours, days, weeks, or even months. It affects the person's response to sound and light, ability to follow commands, speech, and awareness of surroundings. Movies and television often show a person in coma lying very still and quiet as if sleeping and then suddenly waking up and becoming alert. This is not accurate.

No one really knows how much sound, information and activity filter through while a person is in a coma. A person may move or groan and respond to sounds, touch or pain. Family members often believe that the person hears and responds to their voices. These signs may be reflexes - like squeezing a hand or sucking in response to touch. It is hard for families to sort out which responses are reflexive or automatic actions and which are planned or intentional.

A brain injury is usually described as mild, moderate or severe. The length of time that a person is in a coma is one of many factors that determines the severity of an injury.

Brain Injury	Length of coma
▪ Mild	none or very brief
▪ Moderate	up to 24 hours
▪ Severe	more than 24 hours

The length of coma varies for each person because each brain injury is different. Professionals can not predict precisely how long a coma will last. This is frustrating for many families, but the brain is very complicated. Much is still unknown about what happens after it is injured.

Measuring the depth of coma is complicated because there are many levels of awareness and response. It is not as simple as being asleep or awake. The depth of coma can even vary during the day. Examiners can differ in how they evaluate a person's responses to sound, light, touch and commands. Two scales are often used in hospitals and rehabilitation.

Glasgow Coma Scale

This helps medical staff evaluate the level of consciousness. It is based on three measures that each have numbered scores:

- eye opening
- verbal or spoken responses
- motor or physical responses

The overall score has a high of 15. When the score is 13-15, the brain injury is considered *mild;* 9-12 indicates a *moderate* brain injury; 8 or less reflects a *severe* brain injury.

The Glasgow Coma Scale is used with children (ages 4+) and adults.

Rancho Los Amigos Scale

This is a more detailed scale that describes the behaviors and abilities of a person who is gradually coming out of a coma. It is often referred to as the Rancho Scale. It includes 8 levels of response that describe a person's awareness and response to light, sound, touch and commands.

The basic Rancho scale is for children (age 14 years +) and for adults.

Understanding the scales

Ask a doctor or nurse if the Glasgow or Rancho scale has been used to evaluate your relative. If the answer is yes, ask staff:

- to explain what the numbers mean
- if this score has changed since the injury
- what may happen next

Early Stages of Coma Recovery

A person does not just *"wake up"* from a coma. It is a gradual process of becoming more responsive and aware of people and surroundings. Rarely do individuals progress directly through the different levels of consciousness. There is usually some overlap, or back and forth between stages.

Your relative may become confused, not recognize you, talk and behave strangely, swear, become angry, and even be violent. This is a normal stage of coma recovery and it is usually temporary.

Noise, touch, light, and movement may calm or upset the person. Post-traumatic amnesia is common as persons regain consciousness. This means that the person may not remember being hurt and what happened next.

Tips for families to help your relative...

✓ Keep things simple. Do only one activity at a time. Too much talking, noise, touching or activity can confuse the person even more.

✓ Assure your relative that she is safe. Tell her what happened and where she is. Repeat this many times. It may be hard for your relaitve to understand and remember new information.

"You were hit by a roadside bomb in the war.. You are in the hospital."

✓ Tell the person whether it is morning, afternoon or evening. This helps orient your relative to time, but keep it simple.

"It is morning," rather than, "It is eight o'clock."

✓ Let the person know who you are and who is with you.

"This is your wife, Ann. Your Dad is here too."

✓ Touch the person when you speak. This helps your relative figure out where you are, who you

are and what you are doing.

"This is your sister, Kate. I am holding your hand."

✓ Do the same things each time.

"I am going to put some lotion on your legs."

✓ Bring in a favorite item from home. Your relative needs to hear and touch things that are familiar. But again, keep it simple.

"I'm playing your favorite CD of _____."

"I am reading you a card from your daughter."

✓ Avoid arguing. Instead, change the direction or topic of conversation. Your relative may quickly become frustrated and angry, especially when still confused and irritable.

Instead of, "That's not right...," suggest doing something a different way.

✓ Avoid negative or uncomfortable topics. No one knows how much the person hears or understands.

Instead of discussing your relative's condition or upsetting topics by the bedside, go to a private area or separate room.

✓ Avoid asking questions. Describe what is happening or give specific directions.

Instead of, "Can you see me?" say, "I can see you. Your eyes are open."

Instead of, "Can you move your arm?" say, "Try to move your arm."

✓ Give your relative information. Avoid asking, "Do you remember..."

Instead of, "Do you remember the shooting?" say, "You were on foot patrol in Baghdad and were shot. You have been in the hospital for three days."

✓ Help orient your relative with visual information. Post a calendar and mark off each passing day. Bring in family photos or hang favorite pictures on the walls.

✓ Write a short note about your relative and hang it over the bed. This will help nurses, doctors and others know the person better. Describe personal likes and dislikes and include a picture of your relative.

Tips for helping children...

Too often children with a parent or sibling in a coma feel left out and receive little information. Efforts to protect them may increase their fears and anxiety about what has happened to their mother or father, brother or sister.

✓ Ask medical staff for advice on explaining coma to your children.

✓ Use language that your children can understand.

✓ Encourage them to ask questions.

✓ Describe how their parent or sibling looks.

✓ Don't force them to visit until they feel ready - let it be their choice if hospital rules allow it.

✓ Encourage children to send messages by cards, drawings, pictures, or audiotapes.

✓ Call home regularly each day if you are away from home to touch base with your children and to reassure them.

Conclusion

This is a difficult time for everyone in the family. Patience, support, information and help from staff, relatives and friends will help you through this uncertain time.

This article is part of a series on brain injury among children, adolescents and adults. For a free catalog, contact:

Lash & Associates Publishing/Training Inc.
Tel. & Fax (919) 562-0015 or visit our web site
www.lapublishing.com

This article is not intended as a substitute for the medical advice of your physician. Consult your doctor regularly about matters concerning your health, particularly regarding symptoms that require diagnosis or immediate medical attention.

Concussion in Adults

Written by: Ron Savage, Ed.D. & Bill Frey, Ph.D.

✓ recognize concussion symptoms
✓ monitor recovery over time

Concussions are Common

Concussions are the largest group of traumatic brain injuries. They account for almost 70% of all reported traumatic brain injuries. Anyone, any age can experience a concussion... athletes, school teachers, grandmothers, carpenters and service members. Military service member in combat are at high risk for a concussion from explosions, assaults, falls and collisions. A concussion can result from shock waves after a blast or explosion, from a blow to the head, or from a whiplash of the head or neck.

A concussion is a physical injury to the brain that disrupts or interferes with a person's normal functioning. It affects each person differently. For example, some ankle injuries (i.e., sprains and fractures) are more disruptive or limiting to a person's daily routine or lifestyle than others. Likewise, concussions have different consequences for each individual. The better we understand any injury, the better our chances are for a speedier and healthier recovery.

Some concussions cause a person to lose consciousness for a brief period of time – just seconds or minutes. Other concussions do not involve a loss of consciousness. A person may "feel foggy" and have memory difficulties after a concussion without losing consciousness.

Sometimes people have long-term problems after a concussion and do not understand why they are having difficulties.

Concussions and the Brain

A concussion disrupts normal brain function. This may be a temporary inconvenience or it may result in permanent changes. When there are complicating factors, a brain injury can be fatal. All brain injuries must be carefully assessed because of the potential life-threatening danger associated with a brain injury, including a concussion.

CAT scans and MRIs may be used to evaluate a concussion. Measures of physical, cognitive and behavioral responsiveness are also used at the time of the injury to help direct treatment.

Models of what happens to the brain after a concussion indicate that there can be changes in blood flow, brain cell metabolism, neurochemical balance, as well as actual brain cell damage. The severity of a concussion is best determined by the presence of physical and cognitive (memory and thinking efficiency) symptoms over the recovery period.

Recognizing Symptoms and Long Term Effects

Most individual have no long term changes in brain functioning following a concussion. Any cognitive and behavioral changes from the concussion return to normal as the brain repairs itself. This recovery can take days or a few months depending on the biomechanics of the injury and differences among individuals. A person with a concussion can have a wide range of sensory, perceptual, cognitive, emotional and behavioral symptoms during recovery.

Early symptoms include...
- headache
- dizziness or balance problems
- lack of awareness of surroundings (orientation)
- changes in memory and thinking abilities
- tiredness
- vomiting or nausea

Persistent symptoms include...
- headache that won't go away
- lightheadedness
- selective memory and thinking problems
- poor attention and concentration
- changes in sleep habits

- excessive or easy fatigue
- intolerance of bright light or difficulty focusing vision
- intolerance of loud or background noises
- ringing in the ears
- heightened anxiety
- depressed mood
- irritability and low frustration tolerance

It is unusual for a person to have long term effects from a single concussion. However, a person who has more than one concussion, or a series of concussions, may have more complicated symptoms and require more recovery time. A person with long term effects from a concussion needs ongoing medical and psychological support.

Recovery Takes Time

Recovery after a concussion - just like a sprained or fractured ankle - takes time. An initial period of "brain rest" is always important. A person with a broken ankle would not go out the next day and run a marathon. That person likely would take time off work, rest, put the leg up, use crutches, and give the ankle time to recover. Too often after a concussion, a person expects to recover fully in a day or two. Many individuals immediately return to work or school and find themselves unable to think as well and as quickly as they did before. It is not a good idea to "push through" a concussion.

If the person has a second concussion before recovering from the previous concussion, the brain can be more seriously injured. When a person resumes high performance activities like sports or driving too soon, that person is exposed to serious risks of further injury to the brain. This can occur if the athlete returns to the game and is hit again or the person resumes driving a car and has an accident. Doing everyday activities at home, on the job or in school may also alter recovery from a concussion if the person tries to do too much too soon. This can result in longer more complicated recovery time, poor test grades for courses in school, or a poor work evaluation on the job.

See your Primary Care Physician and Specialists

It is important to report a concussion and any changes that you and others notice in your brain functioning to your primary care physician as soon as possible. Just being seen at a hospital emergency department may not be enough. CAT scans and MRI evaluations give limited information for assessing the consequences of a concussion. Some difficulties are not immediately apparent. Your primary care physician can help monitor and manage any changes and refer you to a specialist if further evaluation and treatment are needed.

Neurologists and neuropsychologists specialize in evaluating changes in brain functioning after a concussion. Through testing, a neurologist and a neuropsychologist can help pinpoint a person's problem areas and make recommendations for treatment. They can also give advice on when the person may return to normal work, sports and other activities.

Other specialists may help people understand and adjust to any changes caused by the concussion. Professionals such as psychologists, brain injury counselors, athletic trainers, speech/language pathologists, physical and occupational therapists can help people with more serious concussive symptoms by providing specialized supportive therapies.

Tips on strategies for adjustment after a concussion...

It is important to discuss these strategies with your physician and any specialists after a concussion.

✓ Adjust sleep patterns.
✓ Exercise carefully.
✓ Build rest periods into your schedule.
✓ Reduce workloads.
✓ Allow more time to finish projects.
✓ Develop a written plan to use when you are confused or uncertain.
✓ Use a notebook or calendar to write things down as reminders.
✓ Write down schedules with times, places and persons.
✓ Check off "to do" items as they are completed.
✓ Avoid alcohol or other recreational substances that may slow recovery.
✓ Keep a positive attitude during recovery.

Tips for family members, friends, teachers and employers...

✓ Learn about the symptoms and consequences of concussion.
✓ Help the person make accommodations/adjustments.
✓ Assist in monitoring symptoms.
✓ Ensure that - just like with a broken ankle - the person has ample healing time.

Monitor Symptoms

Keeping track of how you are feeling over the first weeks or months following a concussion can be very helpful. The Post Concussion Checklist makes this an easier task. Before you begin, write down:

1) What happened
2) When you were first treated for the concussion
3) Who first treated you and advice you were given; and
4) How well you followed the advice.

This information should be reported to your physician and other professionals who are treating you.

It is also important to understand that emotional issues associated with the circumstances of a concussion may complicate recovery. Report these feelings to your doctor(s) for more specialized treatments.

References and Resources

Facts about Concussion and Brain Injury. U.S. Dept of Health and Human Services. National Center for Injury Prevention and Control. Atlanta, GA www.cdc.gov/ncipc/tbi/

Frey, WF and Savage, RC (2001). *Journey Toward Understanding Concussion and Mild Traumatic Brain Injury*. Alexandria, VA: Brain Injury Association of America. www.biausa.org.

Giza, CC and Hovda, DA (2001). The Neurometabolic Cascade of Concussion. *Journal of Athletic Training*. Vol. 36 (3): 228-235.

Heads Up: Brain Injury in Your Practice Tool Kit U.S. Dept of Health and Human Services, Centers for Disease Control and Prevention. www.cdc.gov/ncipc/pub-res/tbi_toolkit/toolkit.htm

Hossler, P and Savage, RC (2006). *Getting A-Head of Concussion: Educating the student-athlete's neighborhood*. Wake Forest, NC: Lash and Associates Publishing/Training, Inc.

Ropper, AH and Gorson, KC (2007). Concussion. *The New England Journal of Medicine*. Vol. 356 (2): pp 166-172.

Post-Concussion Check List for Adults

Name: _____ **Family member:** _____

Date of Concussion: _____ **Doctor:** _____

	Week1	2	3	4	5	6	7	8
Sense of Self Rating Rate how close to your normal self you feel now. 10% 25% 50% 75% 90% 100%	%	%	%	%	%	%	%	%
Physical Symptoms **Rate Changes** (none = 0, some = 1, a lot = 2)								
• Headache, dizziness, lightheadedness								
• Vomiting or nausea								
• Numbness or tingling								
• Balance problems, clumsiness, dropping things, tripping often								
• Fatigue, tiring easily, drowsiness								
• Needs extra sleep, or trouble falling or staying asleep								
• Sensitivity to light and noise								
• Blurry vision; different size pupils								
• Ringing in ears								
• Seizures								

If any symptoms persist and/or worsen, contact your primary care physician immediately.

Side 1

Post-Concussion Check List for Adults

Rate Changes (none = 0, some = 1, a lot = 2)	Week1	2	3	4	5	6	7	8
Cognitive and Behavioral Symptoms								
• Is confused, feels in a "fog," has befuddled expression								
• Mixes up time and place								
• Has difficulty with attention or concentration								
• Unable to do more than one thing at a time								
• Does not return to a task if interrupted								
• Has trouble with memory and forgets things								
• Has slurred or irregular speech								
• Takes longer to get things done or complete assignments								
• Has trouble understanding and organizing thoughts or words								
• Is restless, irritable, fussy								
• Acts without thinking								
• Becomes upset easily, loses temper								
• Is sad, has depressed mood								
• Is anxious or nervous								
• Other								

Side 2

Post-Traumatic Headache
Written by: Nathan Zasler, M.D.

✓ recognize causes of headache
✓ understand methods of assessment
✓ manage post-traumatic headache

Headaches after Trauma

The most common physical complaint in up to 70% of all people with a mild brain injury or concussion is headache. It also occurs after more severe brain injury, but is not reported as frequently for some unknown reason. When people seek medical care after a concussion, head trauma or neck whiplash injury, they are often diagnosed with "post-traumatic headache" (PTHA). This is really a catchall phrase. It tells nothing about the headache's cause or how to treat it.

Sources of Head Pain

There are many different sources of head and neck pain, both inside and outside the head. The brain is not a source of pain as it has no feeling. There are many other areas of the body that can cause headaches. Sometimes it is easy to identify and treat these sites. Other times, it is far more complicated.

Your doctor may ask questions about your injury to better understand the cause(s) of your headache. For example, if you were in a car crash, the doctor may question you about seat restraints and the speed of the vehicle. Information will be gathered about any history of direct blows to your head or body and any history of head, neck and whiplash injury. Specifically, your doctor should ask about the presence of the 3 "Cs":

- *cerebral* injury – this means an injury to the brain.
- *cranial* or cranial/adnexal trauma – this means damage to the head/skull and/or structures inside the head such as the mouth, ears and/or sinuses.
- *cervical* injury due to trauma such as whiplash - this can injure muscles, ligaments, nerves and/or blood vessels in the neck.

The Doctor's Evaluation

Your doctor should ask you a number of questions to better understand your headache. Your personal and family history of headache are also important. The major questions that your doctor may ask about your headaches can be expressed in the mnemonic **COLDER**.

This stands for...

Character	what it feels like
Onset	how it starts
Location	where it hurts
Duration	how long it lasts
Exacerbation	what makes it worse
Relief	how it gets better or goes away

There may also be questions about...

- frequency and severity of pain
- other symptoms that go along with your headache
- presence of an aura (sensory changes that typically occur before the headache and are often visual in nature including flashing lights, blind spots, wavy lines, ringing in the ears, bad smells, among others)
- any effects of headaches on daily routine and activities

Your doctor should examine your head, neck, shoulders and any other areas that bother you. Head pain can come from other parts of your body, such as the neck.

A "hands on" assessment by a doctor is crucial to determine the sources of your pain. This may include...

- Inspection - looking
- Palpation - feeling
- Auscultation - using a stethoscope to listen for abnormal body sounds, and
- Percussion - striking or tapping a part of the body with quick, sharp blows and listening for the sounds produced.

The evaluation should also include review of your medical records including x-rays, CT, MRI and any other important tests.

Types of Headaches

There are many different types and causes of headache after a brain, head or neck injury. Because of the medical language in this section, you may not be familiar with all the terms. By reading carefully, they should help you communicate more easily with your doctor.

Musculoskeletal headache

The most common and often most overlooked cause of post-trauma headache is musculoskeletal pain from the neck and cranial/cranial adnexal structures (things in the head but not the brain itself). Musculoskeletal pain is any pain that has its origins from injury to muscles and/or bony structures. The pain will classically be felt in either the head and/or neck. Sometimes pain problems in the neck are actually sent (i.e. referred) into the head and perceived as headache pain.

Musculoskeletal headaches may be caused by a variety of disorders including cervical muscle injury (i.e. strain/sprain). This may develop into a myofascial pain syndrome which can be associated with cervical whiplash injury. Myofascial pain occurs when a muscle develops sensitive areas or "trigger points" that are locally tender when active. Trigger points typically send pain to other areas of the body.

Musculoskeletal headache that is cervicogenic (arising from the neck) usually involves symptoms of pressure and tension, often with a "cap-like" distribution. Here, the headache tends to get worse with stooping, bending or exertion. It may be associated with other symptoms such as dizziness and sensitivity to light and/or sound.

Cervical / cervicogenic headache

This type of headache is very common following trauma. It may be related to problems due to muscle (see above), ligaments, and/or joints (e.g.. facet) injury. Facet joints are located between most verte-

bra of the spine. They act like hinges to help the spine be more flexible. When these joints are damaged, there may be more pressure on the spine and this can cause pain. Treatment may include manual therapies by a therapist, osteopath, chiropractor or a physician trained in manual techniques. A local anesthetic may be injected into the affected facet joint(s) for treatment and/or procedures may be performed to "deaden" nerve in the facet joint on a temporary basis.

If there is instability due to ligament damage from the initial trauma, some clinicians will suggest procedures such as prolotherapy to "tighten" up the connective tissue connections between the joints. More traditional approaches for cervical instability involve surgical management via fusion.

Pain medication may be helpful in controlling cervical headache pain. Physical treatment should be emphasized including manual therapies, massage, strengthening and flexibility exercises, electrical stimulation, and heat/cold therapies.

Temporomandibular joint dysfunction (TMJD)

Commonly known as TMJD, this sometimes occurs after a whiplash injury. It often involves injury to the chewing muscles around the jaw, rather than the jaw itself. However, the jaw joint(s) can be damaged if the muscles cause the bones to grind against one another. TMJD is often over-diagnosed as a result of trauma. Many people have pre-existing TMJD disorders, which may worsen after significant trauma. TMJD is generally treated with prescription anti-inflammatory drugs and muscle relaxants, splints to help realign the jaw, a diet of softer foods, and physical therapy. Surgery is occasionally used to remove damaged tissue, or to implant artificial discs when damage is severe.

Tension type headache

Tension type headaches often feel like a vice gripping the temples. The temples are at the side of the head between the eye and ear. Some people report pain on only one side. It is not clear what triggers this type of headache, although stress and negative emotions are commonly reported. It is even less clear if and how a traumatic brain injury triggers this type of headache.

Treatment of tension headaches usually involves both medication and non-medication approaches. Anti-inflammatory medications are generally prescribed, sometimes along with caffeine, sedatives and/or tranquilizers. Other medications that are sometimes used include selected antidepressants, tizanidine, or botulinum toxin (Botox). Non-medication treatments may include relaxation therapy, EMG biofeedback, cognitive behavioral therapies, stress management, pain management, limited contact treatment and physical therapy.

Neuritic and neuralgic pain

Large nerves in the scalp, face or upper neck may be injured following trauma. This may be the result of direct injury. It may also be caused by pinching of the nerve between muscles in the upper neck that have been injured and are now in a state of "spasm." Sometimes headache pain is caused by small cuts to the scalp that damage the scalp nerves. This type of pain tends to be a shooting, stabbing pain with numbness in the affected scalp area. There are several ways to treat neuritic and neuralgic pain syndromes of the scalp/head. They include local nerve blocks that stop nerve cells from sending pain messages to the brain, treating muscle spasms, electrical stimulation, and acupuncture. There are some medications that a person can apply directly to the painful area of the scalp to decrease pain. In more unresponsive cases, surgery may be needed.

Neurovascular or migraine headache

Post-traumatic neurovascular headache or migraine accounts for about 20% of all chronic post-traumatic headaches. It is generally treated similarly to non-traumatic migraine. Treatment should include looking at all possible factors that may influence the headache picture. This includes reducing "triggers". These may include physical and/or emotional stressors or certain types of food. Birth control pills can also increase migraines for a small percentage of women. Relaxation training and biofeedback are sometimes effective for treating this type of headache. Botulinum toxin injections are sometimes effective, although not FDA approved.

There are other rare causes of headache to consider after a traumatic brain injury and these should be considered if common causes are not found.

Pain Management

Many people with chronic pain develop emotional difficulties. Depression and/or anxiety are common reactions. They may increase a person's sense of pain and distress. A psychologist or pain specialist can help a person with headaches learn how to handle or manage pain. Biofeedback, stress management and cognitive-behavioral therapies have helped many people with headaches. There are professionals, who are skilled at chronic pain management and working with persons with brain injuries and their families, that may help.

Education about post traumatic headache is crucial for treatment success. Understanding the disease process and the expectations of treatment is very important for the individual and family. It is also important to understand how to take prescribed medication and how to avoid side-effects from either under or over usage.

Pain medications may further control post-traumatic pain. Drugs should be used with caution and in particular, opiates and other potentially addicting medications should be used cautiously. Medication side effects can also cause headache as can the overuse of certain types of headache medications such as caffeine, barbiturates, triptans and anti-inflammatory medications. A physician must carefully evaluate these issues.

The pain that is associated with post traumatic headache can interfere with a person's ability to think. It can cause decreased attention, difficulty concentrating and problems remembering. Pain can also cause problems with falling asleep as well as staying asleep which may increase daytime fatigue. Many individuals with significant acute and chronic pain syndromes notice increased irritability and a "shorter fuse" and may even become depressed and/or anxious.

It is possible to successfully manage, if not cure, post traumatic headache and pain in general. It is crucial to help people with chronic pain develop successful adaptive and behavioral skills if treatment for pain management is to be as effective as possible.

Conclusion

When properly treated, most post-traumatic headache is generally not permanent or totally disabling over the long term. However, a very small population will develop post-traumatic headaches that do not respond well to treatment.

It is important to work with your physician to complete thorough pre-injury and post-injury histories and to assure careful clinical evaluation in order to make a proper diagnosis. Be wary of treatment that simply focuses on stopping pain without understanding the reasons for the pain. Most effective treatment strategies involve medical, physical and life management strategies. These help reduce pain as much as possible, guide people in strategies that can help avoid situations that may cause headaches to occur in the future, and help people learn to adapt with chronic pain.

References

Martelli, M.F., Zasler, N.D. (2006). Post-traumatic Pain Disorders: Psychological Assessment and Management. In *Brain Injury Medicine: Principles and Practice*. N. Zasler, D. Katz, R. Zafonte (Eds.). New York: Demos Publishers.

Zasler, N.D., Martelli, M.F. (2006). Post-traumatic Pain Disorders: Medical Assessment and Management. In: Brain Injury Medicine: Principles and Practice. N. Zasler, D. Katz, R. Zafonte (Eds.). New York: Demos Publishers.

Post-Traumatic Stress Disorder PTSD

Written by: Nadia Webb, Psy.D., ABPdN

✓ the causes and symptoms of PTSD in veterans
✓ the effects of PTSD on the brain
✓ treatment of PTSD

What is PTSD?

PTSD is the diagnosis given to individuals with specific psychological symptoms following a traumatic event in their lives. The symptoms of PTSD include...

- intrusive thoughts and memories of the traumatic event (flashbacks)
- emotional numbness
- avoiding reminders of the trauma, and
- hypervigilance (overly alert) to possible dangers.

The symptoms of PTSD may appear after a person is exposed to a traumatic situation where a person fears for their safety or the safety of companions. The traumatic situation typically involves feeling...

- frightened
- horrified or
- helpless to prevent what is happening.

The risk of PTSD increases when a person feels betrayed or deliberately victimized. Other factors that increase the risk are an environment that is unsupportive, blaming or stigmatizing. People with prior histories of abuse or mental health problems are at greater risk.

Crossing the line

Deployment involves exposing yourselves to traumatic situations routinely. Seeing dead bodies is almost universal, and most veterans will have had a close call or known someone who was killed and injured. Almost a quarter of veterans will have sustained serious injuries during combat. The risk of developing PTSD increases with the direct risk to a service member. Only a fraction of service members who experience a trauma will develop PTSD. A person's symptoms have to be so severe that it is hard for the person to function in daily life. The rates of PTSD differ based on where a service member is posted or based. It is estimated that 19% of service members returning from Iraq have PTSD (and 11.3% of service members returning from Afghanistan).

Someone may have many of the symptoms of PTSD during a period or "window" of time after a trauma. If these symptoms fade within the month, it is called an Acute Stress Disorder (ASD) rather than PTSD. For veterans, it is important to know that many of the skills learned during deployment can become almost instinctive and hard to set aside. Quick reflexes and hyper-alertness can be lifesaving during deployment, but swerving to avoid plastic bags or changes in the road texture and difficulty being blocked in at an intersection will cause problems at home.

ASD may fade quickly, but it may also be the first indication of greater distress. It is important not to ignore it. ASD often includes dissociative symptoms, such as "feeling outside my body" or that "things around me are unreal". If the symptoms persist beyond a month, the diagnosis changes to PTSD. Early intervention is important because 75% of people with ASD will go on to develop PTSD.

The PTSD Cycle

PTSD looks different over time because the symptoms tend to wax and wane. PTSD symptoms will typically cycle between intrusive symptoms which disrupt daily life and symptoms that cause feelings of numbness and withdrawal.

Intrusion

Intrusive symptoms include nightmares, "daymares" or flashbacks which feel like the trauma is happening all over again. This may include "seeing" the trauma or feeling the sensations and emotions that accompanied it. In this stage, memories and thoughts about the trauma keep cropping up, making it hard for the person to focus on life or get to sleep at night.

Numbing

The intrusion phases tend to be mixed with periods of numbness. Feelings of being disconnected from life or from family and loved ones may be present when nightmares and intrusive thoughts are not present. People in this phase often feel depressed and empty. Some people respond to these feelings by becoming thrill seekers to feel alive again. However, this can put them at risk for more trauma and head injury. The fear can also trigger flashbacks and a new intrusive phase.

Avoidance

People often begin avoiding any situations or objects that remind them of the accident or traumatic event. Many things can be "triggers" for flashbacks including smells, places, people, weather, etc. As the individual attempts to avoid these triggers, the tragic consequence is that the person's world contracts into a smaller and lonelier place.

Hyperarousal

Regardless of whether they have intrusive or numbing/avoidance symptoms, people with PTSD may startle easily and more dramatically than before. They tend to be anxious and overly vigilant or on the alert to dangers, particularly dangers related to the traumatic event. The worrying may seem out of proportion, even paranoid, to friends and family members. This symptom, by itself, is normal for service members who have recently finished a deployment; it does not mean the service member has PTSD.

PTSD and the Brain

Although PTSD is considered a mental disorder, the stress associated with it can cause physical damage. When stress hormones are at high levels, they become toxic to parts of the brain especially the hippocampus, prefrontal cortex and cerebellum. Each of these regions has an important job to do. The hippocampus is the gatekeeper for factual memories. The prefrontal cortex is involved in planning, judgment and motivation. The cerebellum is involved in fine-tuning motor coordination, learning, and emotional expression. Chronic or under-treated physical pain also boosts stress hormones. Intrusive and hyperarousal symptoms tend to keep stress hormones high.

Can I have PTSD even if I don't remember what happened?

Having little or no memory of the event doesn't prevent PTSD but it makes it less likely. The brain has multiple memory systems. The part of the brain that is the gatekeeper for factual memories (who, what, where and when something happened) is different than the part of the brain that is the gatekeeper for feeling memories. For an individual who experienced an IED explosion, the sound of emergency broadcast tone may leave the person shaken and crying. (IEDs tend to disrupt fluid filled structures in the brain in particular, such as the inner ear, gut, brain, and lungs.)

Treatments

There are many options for treating PTSD. Most people find they need to use a combination of approaches. It is very important to treat it as quickly as possible. PTSD symptoms can become firmly established in an individual and hard to change. The ways that people cope with untreated PTSD tend to make it worse. Untreated PTSD can lead to problems with drug or alcohol abuse, withdrawal, or aggression.

Recovery from PTSD is gradual and often incomplete. Some symptoms may remain, even after treatment, although they are less frequent and less intense. PTSD symptoms that have faded may resurface again after another traumatic event or after another illness or injury. About half of all people with PTSD also experience major depression or problems with drug and alcohol abuse.

What Helps?

Witnessing

Writing about what happened with all the details in the order that they occurred can "anchor" the events and feelings, so that they don't pop up in inappropriate contexts (like flashbacks.) Working with someone to edit and put the story in order is an important part of this. The editor doesn't need to be a mental health professional, just a non-judgmental and supportive person. These stories may be shared with others or kept private.

Counseling

Therapists may help people develop healthier coping strategies and abandon unhealthy ones. They can offer a safe and supportive setting to face fears and decrease sensitivity to triggers associated with PTSD. They can also help address the trauma survivor's feelings of guilt, responsibility and/or rage. Eye Movement Desensitization and Reprocessing (EMDR) is a newer treatment, with some research supporting its usefulness. Many of these interventions can be modified for individuals with brain injury. Most therapists have no training in working with brain injury, but most are willing to consult with a brain injury specialist for guidance.

Medications

Medication effects vary among individuals with PTSD. A wide range of psychiatric medications have proven helpful, although determining which medication will be helpful is hard to do in advance. Usually the SSRI antidepressants, like Zoloft or Prozac, are the starting choices. It is helpful to consult with a neurologist or psychiatrist familiar with brain injury, even if this means traveling to another city. Focusing on competencies and strengths Focusing on competencies and strengths

All trauma survivors carry within themselves the strength that got them through the trauma. Moreover, the trauma was hardly the first difficulty they ever encountered in their lives. What inner strengths have gotten them this far? The answer is different for each person but everyone has inner resources to draw on in troubled times. It is best not to focus exclusively on the problems, difficulties and damage. Rather, it can be helpful to stay focused on the strength that the individual has shown and make it part of the witnessing story being written.

Caring for yourself after a trauma

Sleep

People often put off sleep because of nightmares until they can't stay awake. Or they drink alcohol to "take the edge off." But alcohol disrupts the normal stages of sleep and results in less restorative sleep. Most sleeping pills leave a person feeling groggy the next day. Sleep disruption and sleeping pill hangovers can worsen cognitive difficulties for people with brain injuries. Temporary use of short acting sleeping medications can help during the intrusive phase of PTSD.

Water

It is important to drink a lot of water. Dehydration leaves brain cells more vulnerable to damage from high levels of stress.

Exercise

Stress hormones are part of the "fight or flight" system. They were designed for action, not desk jobs and channel surfing. Physical exercise helps rid the body of these hormones. Feeling healthy can help the person feel more powerful and alive. For service members, who are often young and athletic, finding ways to participated in challenging adaptive sports is often crucial.

Social support

Feeling cared for and feeling like part of a community reduces the level of stress hormones. PTSD or brain injury support groups, therapists, and community support are helpful for individuals and their families.

Relaxation through touch

Massage, stretching, and yoga may reduce stress hormones. They affect deep pressure receptors in the skin and reduce blood pressure, anxiety and physical stress. Stress levels also drop when people pet their animals or watch an aquarium.

Relaxation through mediation or prayer

Scientists who image the brain during meditation or prayer find positive changes in activity level throughout the brain. Both can be very effective in reducing anxiety, decreasing chronic pain, and reducing stress hormones.

Treating chronic pain

Many veterans with PTSD were injured during the traumatic event; IED explosions often cause complex fractures or traumatic amputations, traumatic brain injuries, burns and infections. The complexity of the injuries increases the risk for chronic pain problem. Consider consulting a pain specialist if your pain is disrupting your sleep or daily life activities.

What doesn't help?

Dwelling on it

After a certain point, retelling the story of the trauma isn't helpful. Shift the focus to dealing with life now.

Social isolation

People often retreat from the world after being traumatized. Others vent their anger on family members and close friends, driving away those who love them the most.

Drugs, particularly cocaine and amphetamines.

Research shows that cocaine and amphetamines can increase brain damage. Individuals with brain injury are even more susceptible to the judgment problems, impulsivity, motor problems, and mood swings that drugs and alcohol produce.

Debriefing

Reviewing the events immediately after the trauma is a common practice in disaster work; however, the research doesn't indicate that it helps. Research does show that there are crisis counseling methods that are effective.

Yohimbe or Yohimbine

This herbal supplement is alleged to improve erectile functioning. However, it has been the most reliable drug available to induce flashbacks.

High stress and high drama

Living in a tense, violent or loud neighborhood is not helpful. Nor is participation in criminal activity or high adrenaline recreation. During the numbness phase, people with PTSD often seek out increased risks and stress to feel less deadened. Instead, know that the numbness will pass, while more stress will tend to make the PTSD cycle worse.

Summary

PTSD can be disturbing but temporary if you take the right steps. Reach out to others, including professionals, and make healthier choices day by day. Most people move beyond PTSD, as can you. You won't make all of these changes perfectly, but each change you make will tip the scales toward wellbeing and a more functional life.

References

National Center of PTSD at www.ncptsd.va.gov

National Institute for Mental Health www.nimh.nih.gov/publicat/reliving.cfm

Friedman, M.J., Charney, D.S., Deutch, A.Y. (Eds.) (1995). *Neurobiological and clinical consequences of stress: From normal adaptation to PTSD.* Philadelphia: Lippencott-Raven.

Holeva, V., Tarrier, N., & Wells, A. (2001). Prevalence and predictors of acute stress disorder and PTSD following road traffic accidents: Thought control strategies and social support. *Behavior Therapy, 32,* 65–83.

Hoge, C.W., Auchterlonie, J. L.. Milliken, C. S. (2006). Mental Health Problems, Use of Mental Health Services, and Attrition From Military Service After Returning From Deployment to Iraq or Afghanistan. *JAMA,* 295:1023-1032.

Hoge, C. W., Castro, C. A., Messer, S. C., McGurk, D,., Cotting, D. I., & Koffman, R. L (.2004). Combat Duty in Iraq and Afghanistan, Mental Health Problems, and Barriers to Care. *New England Journal of Medicine.* Vol.351:13-22, No.1.

Undiagnosed Brain Injuries

Written by: Michael P. Mozzoni, Ph.D.BCBA/CBIST. & Marilyn Lash, M.S.W.

✓ recognize signs and symptoms
✓ ask questions and gather information
✓ know what to do and how to seek help

How Many?

The Centers for Disease Control estimates that 5.3 million people in the US - about 2% of the population - live with disabilities from traumatic brain injuries. The majority (85%) of brain injuries are mild and do not result in long-term disabilities, but repeated brain injuries can have cumulative effects. These figures do not include individuals with unidentified brain injuries who are treated and released from emergency departments or seen by local physicians.

Nor do these numbers include brain injuries among troops returning from war zones. While protective equipment in combat areas has reduced the numbers of penetrating head injuries, they can't completely protect the soldier's face, head and neck from all blast injuries. The Defense and Veterans Brain Injury Center (DVBIC) reports that 33% of all soldiers with battle injuries in Operation Iraqi Freedom and Operation have a diagnosis of traumatic brain injury. This is more than double the number seen in past wars.

Brain injuries among soldiers with a loss of consciousness are more readily identified. Soldiers may also have other types of injuries, including burns, missing limbs, internal injuries, lung, ear, nose, sinus and eye injuries. Medics on the battlefield and military hospital units provide emergency trauma care and many are evacuated for further intensive treatment.

It is possible, however, to have a brain injury without a loss of consciousness. Returning soldiers and veterans are at high risk for unidentified brain injuries due to their exposure to blast explosions, land mines, vehicles crashes, falls and gunfire. They may have:

- been thrown off their feet
- knocked to the ground
- felt stunned or confused
- had ringing in the ears or problems hearing
- had trouble breathing
- been hit by flying debris
- been struck by a bullet or fragment

Efforts are underway to increase screening both before and after deployment for possible brain injuries at military bases and among National Guard and Reserves Units.

Making the Diagnosis

Diagnosing a mild brain injury (often called a concussion) is often difficult or delayed because neurological tests may not show any abnormalities. The diagnosis may be missed during the service member's deployment. Or it may be ignored or overlooked by the solider because the symptoms seem minor compared to the more severe injuries among comrades. Also some service members prefer not to report their injury as they may want to stay with their comrades or wish to avoid delaying their return home via the medical hospital in Germany. Many service members and civilians do not even seek medical treatment after a blow to the head, believing that any changes are temporary or not serious.

One of the hallmarks for determining the severity of a brain injury is coma. Individuals with a mild brain injury or concussion may not seek treatment immediately, since they either do not lose consciousness or do so for only seconds or minutes. But even a "mild" brain injury can have short-term and/or long-term consequences. It is not necessary to have lost consciousness for an injury to the brain to occur. It is frequently the case, in undiagnosed brain injuries, that the person has had several "mild" (grade 1) concussions. The person may report only an ear ache or cracked teeth following a blast. All persons with blast related traumatic brain injury have ear injuries but not all ear injuries indicate a traumatic brain injury. However, it is a powerful marker that should be followed-up.

Signs after coming home

Many people with undiagnosed brain injuries return to work after a car crash or fall and find it difficult to concentrate, stay alert and handle multiple tasks. Many risk losing their jobs or are fired, but still can't identify the cause of their difficulties. Others, injured as youth, never develop job skills and have trouble finding or holding a job. Most vocational failures are caused by memory and attentional disorders, poor social skills, poor self-awareness, disinhibition, low initiative, and alcohol abuse.

As service members and veterans return home and resume life on base or in the community, they may find themselves having new difficulties "picking up when they left off" and "getting back on track." There can be many physical and emotional reasons for this as exposure to war changes a person as a result of sustained stress. It can be hard to "fit in" once back home. There may be new pressures with finances, family, and careers. A mild to moderate traumatic brain injury can also mimic Post Traumatic Stress Syndrome (PTSD) with short attention span, restricted emotional range and memory difficulties. It may be difficult for the returning service member to resume as the loving, attentive and sensitive spouse. It is important to be aware of the possibility that an undiagnosed brain injury may be contributing to these difficulties.

New Risks

Many people start using alcohol or drink more after a brain injury. Others stop for a while, but begin again later. Persons with brain injuries are at increased risk for addictive behaviors if they rely on substances for coping, alertness or socialization.

Some adults find that alcohol now has increased effects. Their behaviors alienate friends and family and risk repeated brain injuries. Others are arrested for disorderly conduct, driving while intoxicated or assaults.

Previous tendencies toward violence may be greater after a brain injury. Even a previously non-violent individual may have difficulty with anger and violence if certain areas of the brain are affected. Poor anger control is heightened by alcohol after a brain injury. Many prisoners convicted of violent criminal acts have histories of unrecognized and mistreated brain injuries.

Repeated injuries

Impulsivity (acting before thinking), and poor judgment increase the risk for further injury or legal encounters. Brain injury is a risk factor for another brain injury when people think they have recovered (poor awareness) and resume risky behaviors. This is a factor in sports related injuries when a player returns to the game too soon. This player is vulnerable to Second Impact Syndrome, which can result in a more serious injury and even death. A person with a brain injury is three times more likely to have a second brain injury due to resumption of risky behavior and impaired safety judgment, especially when alcohol is used.

Inappropriate treatment

I just don't feel like myself...it's as though I'm in a fog.

I went back to work, but I'm just getting further behind.

I must be going crazy... something's wrong but I don't know what.

These are typical comments by individuals and service members with undiagnosed brain injuries and illustrate their confusion, worry and frustration. Accurate diagnosis is the key to understanding changes, providing emotional supports and developing compensatory strategies. A traumatic brain injury that is diagnosed as PTSD may be especially difficult as one or both may be present.

Deciding how to direct treatment may not be as obvious as the behaviors. Without medical records to review, behaviors are too often viewed as delinquent, psychiatric or the result of PTSD. Students with brain injuries are too often inappropriately classified as having an emotional disorder, attention deficit disorder or learning disability. Adolescents and adults may struggle with substance abuse or face criminal charges or homelessness. Mental health professionals unfamiliar with brain injuries may miss opportunities for accurate diagnosis.

Many disturbances of mood and behavior related to a brain injury result in an inappropriate and ineffective psychiatric treatment model. This squanders limited resources and results in poor outcomes with frequent readmissions to psychiatric, juvenile detention, or criminal facilities.

Questions to Ask

- Has the person had a blow to the head, exposure to a blast, toxins, or diseases of the central nervous system?

    It is not necessary to have lost consciousness for an injury to the brain to occur. It is frequently the case, in undiagnosed brain injuries, that the person has had several "mild" (grade 1) concussions.

- If the person has been exposed to a blast ask:
    - ☐ Did you rupture an ear drum?
    - ☐ Did you have heavy nose bleeding after the blast?
    - ☐ Did you have difficulty breathing, and if so for how long?
    - ☐ Were you struck by debris? If so, where?
    - ☐ Were you knocked down or thrown as a result?
    - ☐ Did you feel dazed or stunned after the blast?
    - ☐ Did you see a friend killed or maimed in the blast?

- Ask the person to show you any scars, especially on the head and face. Ask permission to feel the person's head and examine any "dings or dents".

- Ask how the injury happened and if there are any scars not visible. Ask questions about injures several different ways, such as...
    - ☐ Have you ever been in a car crash?
    - ☐ Have you ever felt dazed or stunned after a fall?
    - ☐ Have you ever been hit in the head during a fight or playing sports?

- Check to see if there is any record or indication of abuse or beating by asking if the person has been:
    - ☐ punched
    - ☐ beaten with a stick, board, pipe, or belt buckle
    - ☐ beaten with a belt or switch other than on the buttocks
    - ☐ been deliberately cut, burned, or thrown down stairs or across a room.

- Has the person been abused? Get the "story" concerning scars and psychopathology in the family?

- Does the person, or any first degree relatives, have a history of psychiatric hospitalization or extreme violence within the family?

What to Look For

Family members and professionals can use the following checklist to identify and difficulties or changes. This information should be shared with a physician to help determine if a brain injury or concussion may have occurred.

Things to observe

- ✓ Note problems, especially difficulty in thinking and short term memory, such as saying months of the year backwards (Dec-Nov-Oct), recalling word lists with immediate recall, then delayed 5 minutes.
- ✓ Assess the person's strength and speed.
- ✓ Assess whether strength and speed differ significantly between left and right sides.
- ✓ Look for problems with coordination or balance.
- ✓ Notice whether the person self discloses too much for the situation.
- ✓ Recognize difficulty making small talk.
- ✓ Observe whether the persons maintains personal space.
- ✓ Assess whether the person is overly self-focused or paranoid.
- ✓ Note if the person has difficulty staying on topic or maintaining a conversation.
- ✓ Note word finding problems or novel word use.

Checklist of Signs and symptoms

Changes in how a person moves, thinks, acts, and communicates are warning signs. Use these checklists to gather information to discuss with a doctor.

Physical changes – *are there…*
- ☐ changes in how the person walks or moves (slower, faster, awkwardly, etc.)
- ☐ problems with balance
- ☐ poor coordination
- ☐ muscles that appear too tense or flaccid
- ☐ marks, scars, or dent near and on the head
- ☐ frequent headaches
- ☐ history of seizures
- ☐ decreased strength and endurance
- ☐ significant differences in left/right strength and speed
- ☐ problems with hearing
- ☐ problems with sense of smell

Cognitive changes – *is there...*
- ☐ difficulty with memory
- ☐ shorter attention span

Does the person have less...
- ☐ insight
- ☐ judgment
- ☐ reasoning
- ☐ sound decision making
- ☐ generalization of skills
- ☐ range of emotions
- ☐ awareness of other's emotions

Does the person have difficulties with...
- ☐ acquiring new skills
- ☐ learning new information (especially verbal)
- ☐ processing and manipulating information
- ☐ following verbal and written directions
- ☐ speech impairments, i.e. word finding and articulation errors

Behavioral problems - Does the person have...
- ☐ less control and more aggression
- ☐ shorter fuse
- ☐ poor persistence or stick to it-ness
- ☐ property destruction
- ☐ low frustration level
- ☐ impulsive actions
- ☐ disinhibited (says/does whatever comes to mind)
- ☐ decreased motivation
- ☐ socially inappropriate comments or actions
- ☐ immature behavior
- ☐ depressive episodes
- ☐ egocentric or self-centered behavior
- ☐ reports recurring nightmares/troublesome thoughts
- ☐ non-compliant (won't follow rules, instructions, or directions)

Social problems- *Does the person have...*
- ☐ poor eye contact
- ☐ inability to stay on topic
- ☐ poor personal hygiene
- ☐ excessive self focus
- ☐ "loner" life style
- ☐ paranoid behavior
- ☐ sexual acting out behavior
- ☐ invasion of personal space of others
- ☐ inability to initiate and maintain small talk

- ☐ socially inappropriate statements
- ☐ poor regulation of self disclosure (shares too much about self for the situation)
- ☐ inability to form long-term intimate relationships

What to do if you suspect there is a brain injury
If the person scores at least one item in each category above, a brain injury may be indicated.

✓ Contact your VA Hospital/Clinic and ask for a Traumatic Brain Injury (TBI) Screening.

✓ Seek a referral for neuropsychological testing. Choose a neuropsychologist familiar with mental health and combat issues, vocational rehabilitation, and substance abuse,.

✓ Obtain complete medical and psychiatric history, including neurodiagnostic evaluations, i.e., CTs, MRIs, EEGs, neuropsychological tests and behavioral assessments.

✓ Learn about educational and support programs designed for returning troops through the VA, National Guard, or military bases.

✓ Consider referral for treatment, either out-patient rehabilitation, day treatment, in-patient rehabilitation or individualized sessions for cognitive/behavioral remediation.

✓ Be sure the program or professionals specialize in brain injury rehabilitation.

✓ Bring a list of all medications (including vitamin supplements) to the attention of all treating physicians.

Treatment of a person with a traumatic brain injury is a family affair. Everyone involved with the person needs to participate.

Conclusion
While the severity of a brain injury can be categorized as "minor", individuals still may have changes affecting cognition (attention, concentration, and memory), affect (depression, anxiety and irritability), and somatic changes (headache, dizziness, fatigue, difficulty sleeping, and sensory impairments).

Mild brain injury typically does not cause prolonged impairments. Most people recover within three months. However, 15% of those with mild brain injuries may have persistent symptoms in the form of post-concussion syndrome. Accurate diagnosis is critical for providing treatment by experienced professionals, giving emotional support, and developing long term coping strategies.

References

American Academy of Neurology (1997). *Practice parameter: The management of concussion in sports* (summary statement). Neurology; 48:581-585.

Jacobs,HE. Iatrogenesis (1998). *Brain Injury Source*; 2(3):26-27,50.

Langley MJ, & Kiley DJ (1992). Prevention of substance abuse in persons with neurological disabilities. *NeuroRehbilitation*; 2(1):52-64.

Lewin ICF (1992). *The cost of disorders of the brain*. Washington, DC: National Foundation for the Brain.

Lewis, DO., Moy E., Jackson LD., Aaronson R., Restifo N., Serra S., Simos A (1985). Biopsychosocial characteristics of children who later murder: A prospective study. *American Journal of Psychiatry*; 142:10:1161-1167.

Mozzoni, M.P. (1997). Rehabilitating brain injured children. *Case Review*; 22-23, 84.

3 Questions DVBIC TBI Screening Tool. www.DVBIC.org

Guide to Medications

After Brain Injury
Written by: Peter Patrick, Ph.D.

✓ understand reasons for medication
✓ identify benefits and side effects
✓ discuss medication with a doctor

Why Take Medication?

Medications may help a person with a brain injury. They may be used to treat some of the physical, emotional and cognitive effects of a brain injury. It is important for individuals and families to learn about the use, side effects and interactions of any medications.

Emotional and psychological changes

There are many changes and struggles in a person's life after a brain injury. Adjusting to changes in abilities and opportunities can be hard. People often feel depressed, anxious, frustrated, or angry after a brain injury. They may have difficulty controlling emotions and have less control over their feelings. Some people even have personality changes and different temperaments after a brain injury.

These feelings usually surface after a person leaves the hospital and has returned home. Families often use the words "like a different person now" to describe how much the person has changed. The person may find it hard to return to school or work, keep friends, and keep up with the pace and demands of daily life. It can take a long time for a person to recover from a brain injury. The person may never be the same as before the injury. This can be very difficult for everyone in the family.

The emotional and psychological changes in a person after a brain injury can be confusing, frightening and worrisome for the entire family. Many families report that these changes are harder to deal with than any physical changes. Emotional changes - small and large - can affect a person's recovery and progress. They can occur for many reasons.

Changes in the brain

Damaged areas of the brain may no longer work as well as before the injury. Mild to moderate brain injuries are often not detected in an MRI or CT examination. There can be changes in the brain at the microscopic or chemical level that do not show on the MRI or CT scan. Brain chemistry affects how a person feels, thinks and behaves.

A brain injury may affect the chemicals in the brain that help regulate or control a person's mood and emotions. These chemicals may be produced in smaller or larger amounts after a brain injury. They may even affect the person differently after a brain injury. Careful use of medication can help restore chemical balances in the brain.

The brain has something called "receptors". These are nerve cells that respond to drugs and nutrients. The receptors may react differently after a brain injury. They can become more or less sensitive and change how a person reacts or feels.

Some people with brain injuries become more or less sensitive to common over the counter medications such as aspirin, vitamins, and cold remedies. They can be more sensitive to their side-effects. Some people are even more sensitive to caffeine after a brain injury.

There are many different ways to help people with the psychological and emotional challenges after a brain injury. Counseling and psychotherapy are usually suggested before trying medication. This is especially true for children and adolescents. Sometimes medications are used along with counseling or therapy. Medication is usually not the first choice for emotional help. Exceptions are extreme cases where a person is very aggressive, deeply depressed or psychotic.

Improving cognitive abilities

Using medications during the early treatment of a brain injury can be helpful. By increasing mental awareness and alertness, the person may be more able to participate in a rehabilitation program. There are medications that help some people improve attention, concentration and mental endurance on a long-term basis. Other newer medications are showing promise in improving memory, decision-making, problem solving and other executive skills. This work is still in the early stages of development.

Attitudes and Beliefs about Using Medication

Many factors affect a person's decision to take medication. People have many attitudes or beliefs about using medication. Some people prefer to use medication only for physical ailments. Others believe that medication can be used to help a person deal with emotional stress. It is important that everyone involved in the individual's care understand how the person feels about using medication. Everyone must be clear about why a person may or may not need medication.

Cultural, religious, social and personal beliefs can also affect this decision. Some people feel fortunate to know that something is available to help with a difficult problem. Others feel that taking medication is a crutch or a sign of weakness. Some feel that using medication decreases their independence and increases their dependency on things outside the body. Still other people equate taking prescribed medications with illicit drugs, worry about addiction, or developing other illnesses such as cancer. Others may only want "natural" things in their bodies. Even the cost of medications is a factor.

It is important for individuals to express their personal beliefs about the use of medications and to listen to the beliefs of others. Talking this over with a doctor and other qualified people is essential.

Effective use of medication is not an on-again, off-again decision or process. There are four major phases of treatment:

- *Preparatory phase*
  The person learns about medication options and reviews concerns. This is the time to identify specific goals and outcomes from treatment.

- *Beginning medication treatment*
  Initial effects of treatment are evaluated.

- *Initial adjustments*
  Dosages and medications may be varied to reach treatment goals.

- *Ongoing management*

Continuing effects of medication are evaluated. The person and the doctor talk about the need for treatment and whether it will be ending or continue.

Talking with the Doctor

The relationship with a doctor, or whoever is prescribing drugs, is critical. It is very important that this person (the prescriber) have experience treating persons with brain injury. Many medications and common doses of medication may not work the same after a person has a brain injury. They may even have the opposite effect than intended. For example, a medication intended to calm a person may increase agitation after a brain injury.

Prescribers have different experience and training. The amount of time they have to meet and talk with patients varies. It is important that a person with a brain injury feels comfortable with who is providing care - whether it is a physician, nurse practitioner or physician assistant. Ask questions about their experience and knowledge about the uses of medications after brain injury. Ask how and when they are available to answer questions and discuss concerns. If not satisfied, ask the primary physician for a recommendation of someone with the time and experience needed.

Finding the right medications and doses can take time and repeated efforts because each brain injury is different. The person with a brain injury and the doctor must consider whether the medication is...

- helping the person be more successful in daily life
- covering up other symptoms, or
- having a negative effect.

Good medication management should contribute to a quality of life and not worsen a person's condition.

Managing Side Effects

Side effects are unintended consequences of medications. They can occur for many reasons. Most medications have some side effects, but they are usually manageable and only affect a small percentage of people. Medication is only continued in these cases when the benefits of the treatment far outweigh the side effects and when side effects are not likely to cause more serious problems.

It is important to learn to identify these effects in order to manage them properly. Some side effects can be serious. Others are only irritants and need not require stopping the medication. The doctor may change the dosage or time schedule to manage some side effects.

Side effects can occur when the medication affects other areas of the brain or other parts of the body. Most medications are not precise enough to affect just one specific area. There can be physical side effects such as changes in blood pressure or heart rate. Seizures can even be a side effect. Other side effects can cause changes in mental function, balance, coordination, mental endurance, or even changes in memory and learning. A person may become sleepy or tired. Some side effects may be unique to the individual taking the drug.

Allergic reactions are different from side effects to a medication. Allergic reactions can occur with the person's first exposure to the drug. They can be serious and require immediate medical attention for the person. Other allergic reactions can occur over time as the body builds up a reaction to the medication. This can also happen with re-exposure to a drug. Typically, allergic reactions are serious and usually mean that the person is not able to take the medication.

Managing Drug Interactions

Medications can interact with one another. This can cause unintended effects. It is important for the doctor to know what other medications a person is taking. This includes over the counter medications, as well as herbal remedies or "natural" supplements. Many natural supplements have a variety of active agents. Many supplements have not been fully tested in scientific studies.

Medications can compete with one another for absorption in the stomach or small intestines. They can also affect each other as they are broken down and distributed in the body.

Some medications can raise or lower the levels of other medications. This can have the effect of increasing or decreasing the dose of other medications. For example, taking a new medication that lowers the therapeutic level of an anti-seizure medication can increase the chance of the person having a seizure.

Lessons Learned
Tips on using medications...

✓ Find a doctor or clinician able to prescribe who is skilled and familiar with the use of medications following brain injury. Make sure that this is a person you can trust and have a good working relationship with.

✓ Consider your response, side effects and interactions when deciding which medication is best for you.

✓ Learn about possible side effects and drug interactions. Most side effects are manageable and are best controlled when you have an active working relationship with your doctor or clinician. Some side effects or interactions can be serious if not detected early.

✓ Take time to learn about your condition and to set up a program with your doctor or nurse. Once medications are started, communicate with the clinician who prescribes your medication.

✓ Identify specific factors for measuring success or failure in your medication use.

✓ Realize that taking medications requires your active involvement and participation.

✓ Discuss problems with your medication with your prescriber, especially when you think it is not working or causing side effects.

✓ Medications seldom work alone. Additional therapy, family education or management plans are needed for the best results.

Your Checklist Before Beginning Medication
Tips on questions to ask...

✓ What is the medication for?

✓ What is the dose?

✓ What improvement should you watch for?

✓ What side effects and interactions should you be aware of?

✓ Is there a plan with your doctor for monitoring use?

References

Stahl, SM. (2005). *Essential Psychopharmacology: The Prescriber's Guide.* New York, NY: Cambridge University Press.

Bezchlibnyk-Butler, KZ, & Virani, AD. (2004). *Clinical Handbood of Psychotropic Drugs for Children and Adolescents.* Ashland, OH: Hogrefe & Huber Publishers.

Stein, D, Lerer, B, & Stahl, S. (2005). *Evidence-based Psychopharmacology.* New York, NY: Cambridge University Press.

How Medications Work
After Brain Injury
Written by: Peter Patrick, Ph.D.

✓ understand the effects of medications
✓ talk with the doctor about medications

Medications for Psychological Recovery

Medications are used to treat many different illnesses, emotions and conditions. We often take them without thinking too much about how they work, just as long as they do the job. People are often confused about using medications after a brain injury, especially those that affect how we think, feel, or act. How does a medication reverse symptoms of depression, anxiety or memory disturbance?

Inside Your Brain

Your brain has billions of nerve cells. They control how you think, move, act, and manage everything you do. Different nerve cells control different abilities such as talking, emotional reactions, moving, thinking, and so on. Nerve cells communicate with one another by sending chemicals, known as neurotransmitters, to other nerve cells.

There are receptors on the surface of each nerve cell that are sensitive to specific neurotransmitters. The neurotransmitters are messengers. Receptors receive the message.

There are different neurotransmitters for different functions. The neurotransmitters and receptors act much like a key and lock. When the key (the neurotransmitter) fits the lock (nerve cell receptor), that nerve cell reacts. Put simply, this is how nerve cells "talk" to one another.

Your Brain after an Injury

We now know that there are changes in nerve cells, receptors and neurotransmitters after a brain injury or illness. Nerve cells and receptors are often damaged or destroyed as a result of an illness or injury. This can disrupt the balance in the types of nerve cells and receptors in your brain. This can affect how you think, act and feel. Your brain's ability to make the neurotransmitters that your nerve cells need to communicate with each other can change. Your brain may start producing too little or too much of different neurotransmitters. This too will affect how you think, act and feel.

Restoring the Balance

Sometimes parts of your brain will recover and restore some of the balance of nerve cells and neurotransmitters. Other times, treatment and therapies are needed.

People's brains change as they learn or are trained. This is why rehabilitation therapies are so important. For example, physical therapy actually gets nerve cells to form new networks in your brain to improve how you walk. Similar changes have been discovered after therapy, counseling and education.

Active learning and therapies are often not enough to restore balance to the brain. Medication can help. When properly used, medications can help improve or return balance to the neurotransmitters and nerve cells in your brain. Proper medication management is not as simple as taking a pill.

There are many things to consider including:
• how your body reacts to medication
• how medication affects your brain
• medication interactions, and
• how precisely medications restore balance to nerve cells and neurotransmitters.

The Body's Reaction to Medication

Your body reacts to each medication you take. The technical terms are:
• Absorption - how medication enters the blood stream
• Distribution - how medication is sent through the body
• Metabolism - how medication is broken down and changed in the body
• Elimination - how the body removes medication

Each step can be affected by changes in health, nutrition and other medications.

Absorption

Most medications are absorbed in your small intestine. Some can be directly injected into your blood stream, or absorbed in the mouth, stomach or lungs. They then circulate in the blood stream, attached to proteins for transportation. The part that is not attached circulates freely. The unattached medication is available for therapy. Medication that is not bound to proteins enters your brain.

Distribution

Portions of each dose of medication begin to build up in the body and penetrate tissues with repeated doses over time. While we may want the medication to penetrate brain cells only, most other body tissues are also penetrated. As the medication builds up in your body, it eventually crosses a protective barrier between the blood in the rest of your body and your brain. It then begins to affect the brain's neurotransmitters and nerve cells.

Metabolism and Elimination

The first thing our body tries to do when we take a new medication is to break it down and eliminate it. This is a protective response to anything foreign that enters your body. Medications are initially seen as foreign agents. Most medications first pass through the liver where they are broken down and eliminated through the kidneys. Some bypass the liver and are directly eliminated by the kidneys.

Effects on the Brain and Body

Medications can have many different effects including therapeutic effects, side effects and interactions.

Medication Therapeutic Effects

Therapeutic effect is the desired clinical change that helps a person reduce suffering and/or improve overall well-being. This happens when the nerve cells in the brain communicate with each other better because of the medication.

We already explained that nerve cells generally communicate with one another by releasing neurotransmitters between one another. When the key (neurotransmitter) fits the lock (nerve cell receptor), it causes that nerve cell to react. Medication can increase, decrease, or stop the nerve cell's response. This affects our actions.

Medication can change the way that nerve cells communicate to one another by:

- turning nerve cells on or off
- increasing or decreasing neurotransmitters in the brain
- blocking or changing the sensitivity of a nerve cell's receptors.

Different neurotransmitters have different effects on brain cells. Some of the more common neurotransmitters include:

Serotonin eases chronic anxiety and depression.

Norepinepherine treats depression and various forms of anxiety.

Epinephrine activates people and our "fight or flight" response.

Dopamine affects movement and our sense of reward.

Glutamate is important in learning and nerve activation.

Gaba is important in relaxation, prevention of seizures and acute management of anxiety.

Acetylcholine helps movement and learning.

How Medications Affect Nerve Cells and Neurotransmitters

There are many different ways that medications create these changes.

Help release a neurotransmitter

Some medications help the nerve cell release more of a neurotransmitter. This affects behavior. Amphetamine and Ritalin are two examples of medications that promote release.

Re-uptake blocking

Some medications build up the effect of a neurotransmitter by blocking its re-absorption into the cell. This creates a larger pool of the neurotransmitter near the receptors of other nerve cells. This increases its effect. Prozac, Paxil and Zoloft are common medications that work this way.

Produce more neurotransmitter

Sometimes the medication helps the cell make more neurotransmitter. This can also increase its effect. L-dopa and Sinemet are examples.

Direct effect

Sometimes medication acts just like a neurotransmitter. This causes other nerve cells to react without increasing the brain's production of a neurotransmitter. Bromocriptnine and Mirapex are examples.

Receptor blockade

Some medications block cell receptors to specific neurotransmitters. This decreases the cell's overall responsiveness, or it makes it more receptive to another neurotransmitter. This is called cross blocking. Risperidone, Zyprexa and newer antipsychotics are examples of this.

Receptor modification

The number of receptors on the surface of a cell can be changed by medications. When medication increases the number of receptors, it is called up-regulation. When it decreases the number of receptors, it down-regulates the cell. This results in an increase or decrease in cell activity.

Medication Side Effects

We may only want to change the way that nerve cells and receptors in the brain respond to medications and neurotransmitters. However, most medications also affect other parts of the body. This can cause unintended side effects. For example, serotonin is a neurotransmitter that is increased by the medications Prozac, Paxil, or Zoloft. Increased serotonin can help lift depression and make people feel better. However, these medications can also affect serotonin receptors in other areas of the brain, such as the hypothalamus and cause nausea. They can affect receptors in the stomach and create gastrointestinal discomfort. Serotonin receptors are also found on the platelets in your blood and in your lungs. This can result in some people bruising more easily.

Minor medication side effects are often managed by changing the dose or the time it is taken. More serious side effects may require discontinuing the medication or taking additional medication to help balance and reduce side effects. Physical symptoms of side effects can include changes in heart rate, blood pressure or blood chemistry. Side effects on mental well-being can alter concentration, speed of responsiveness or even memory. That is why it is so important to work closely with your doctor.

Medication Interactions

Other medications, nutritional or herbal products, or even some foods can easily change a medication's effects. Just because something is labeled herbal or natural does not mean that it is safe. Some supplements have not been properly tested. Some are very powerful. They may affect prescribed medications.

Medication interactions can begin as soon as you take a drug. For example, swallowing multiple medications with certain nutrients can cause them to compete with each other for entry into your blood stream. Drinking grapefruit juice when taking Buspar can actually increase the absorption of the medication by your body and its effect. Other foods or supplements can block or increase intended effects.

Most importantly, medications can affect enzymes in the liver. These enzymes break down and metabolize the medication so it is eliminated from your body. Certain medications can slow down this process, while others quicken it. This can have the same effect as changing the medication dosage. For example, some antiseizure medications quicken the breakdown of some of the new antidepressants. This results in the brain receiving less of the dosage and makes it a less effective anti-depressant.

Knowing how your medication interacts with other substances is important so that both you and your doctor understand how the drug is affecting you.

Using Your New Knowledge

Medication management requires everyone to closely monitor effects and to know what to expect from the treatment. Medications can help greatly when the right medication is matched to the right problem. It is also important to understand how medications interact with your overall health, nutrition, sleep, other medications, and events in your daily life.

It is important to ask questions and to encourage your doctor or nurse to take time to explain things to you. With your new knowledge, you will be better able to ask questions and understand their explanations.

It is important to read this tip card several times and to show it to your doctor for more instruction. It is also important to look at specific sections as you begin to use a medication, after you have been on the medication for some time, and if you are considering discontinuing it. Recovery following brain injury is a long term process. This new knowledge can help you make the best recovery possible.

Tips for lessons learned...
✓ Medications produce results by affecting brain chemistry.
✓ Medications are both affected by the body (pharmacokinetics) and affect the body (pharmacodynamics).

✔ Medications can have unintended side effects that must be monitored.
✔ Most side effects are mild, but some people may be overly sensitive to these effects. That is the reason that many medications are controlled by prescription.
✔ Medications can interact with other medications, over the counter drugs, supplements, foods and other things that you consume.
✔ Knowing how medications work can better prepare you to monitor medication that you and others use.

References

Julien, R. M. (2005). *A Primer of Drug Action*, 10th edition. New York, NY: Worth Publishers.

Stahl, S. (2000). *Essential Psychopharmacology: Neuroscientific Basis and Practice Application,* 2nd edition. New York, NY: Cambridge Press.

Communicating with an Adult

After Brain Injury

Written by: Roberta DePompei, Ph.D. & Marilyn Lash, M.S.W.

✓ describes changes in communication
✓ shows how to improve communication

Introduction

Reading, writing, speaking, conversing, gesturing – any of these can be affected when a person has a brain injury. Changes in a person's speech, language, or thinking can make it harder for a person with a brain injury to learn, have conversations and join social outings. This can result in a communication disorder.

Important definitions

Communication: Methods that people use to understand an idea or express a thought include listening, speaking, reading, writing, and gesturing.

Speech: This is the production of sounds that make up words and sentences.

Language: Language skills are different from speech skills. Language is the use of words and sentences to understand, convey or express ideas.

Cognitive-Communication: This term refers to the use of language with the skills needed for thinking and learning. Cognitive-communication skills are the use of language along with attention, memory, self-awareness, organization, problem solving, and reasoning to communicate effectively. They help us think and learn.

How Does a Brain Injury Affect Communication?

An injury can affect areas of the brain that control producing speech, understanding what is said, or using words to make sentences and express ideas. This affects communication. Changes can lead to loss of friends, misunderstandings, or poor performance in school or on the job. The person with a communication disorder may feel frustrated, lonely, angry or depressed.

How can speech be affected?

Most individuals regain the ability to produce the sounds of speech and words after a brain injury. These skills usually improve as the person physically recovers. But it is more complex when the person has difficulties with paralysis, swallowing, or other types of motor incoordination.

Motor incoordination (muscles that do not move smoothly to produce clear speech) can include dysarthria and apraxia. Dysarthria is a term used to describe speech that is unclear. This is because the motor/muscle control of the tongue, jaw, and lips does not work together. Apraxia is a term used to describe speech that is unclear but the muscle/motor control of the tongue, jaw and lips is normal. The speech is distorted because messages from the brain to the mouth are inadequate and clear speech is not produced.

Characteristics of unclear speech may include:

- slurred words
- drooling
- difficulty swallowing
- hoarse or nasal voice
- slow speech or fast speech or
- total loss of verbal speech.

What Are Language Problems?

There are two types of language abilities to consider. The checklists will help you gather information about a person's use of language. Share this with therapists, physicians and family members.

Receptive skills

This is the ability to understand what is said or written. Use the lists below and check the box that applies to you or your family member. Signs of changes in receptive language are difficulty with...

	often	some	never
Recognizing words	☐	☐	☐
Keeping up with the rate, complexity, or amount of spoken or written information	☐	☐	☐
Requesting information be repeated several times	☐	☐	☐
Paying attention in conversations or in class	☐	☐	☐
Understanding or recalling what was read	☐	☐	☐
Remembering instructions or following directions.	☐	☐	☐

A person with a brain injury may also have a hearing loss. A decrease in hearing can cause the above behaviors or symptoms. It is important to have a complete hearing test by an audiologist to rule out a hearing loss before questioning receptive language.

Expressive skills

This is the ability to speak or write. As a person recovers from a brain injury, most receptive and expressive language skills that are needed for routine communication may appear normal or close to normal. Rarely will there be a problem with putting a sentence together or understanding everyday language. It is the more subtle problems with language and cognitive-communication that are often overlooked.

Signs of changes with expressive language include when a person...

	often	some	never
Has a hard time remembering a word when speaking or writing	☐	☐	☐
Uses rude or immature language	☐	☐	☐
Has problems developing and using new vocabulary	☐	☐	☐
Talks about unrelated topics	☐	☐	☐
Fails to use proper "social graces" in situations	☐	☐	☐
Makes up stories or explanations for situations	☐	☐	☐
Uses hyperverbal or rapid non-stop talking	☐	☐	☐
Gives lengthy unorganized explanations	☐	☐	☐
Retells the same story over and over	☐	☐	☐
Has difficulty writing sentences	☐	☐	☐
Has trouble spelling words correctly.	☐	☐	☐

Are there tests to find problems with language?

Standard tests often do not find major problems with language in a person with a brain injury. The individual may look better on the test than in actual daily life. This is why it is important for family members to report any changes in communication that are causing difficulties.

What Types of Cognitive Communication Problems Can Exist?

Many individuals with brain injury appear to have little difficulty with language skills, particularly in non-stressful situations. However, use of language may lessen or fall apart when the stress of communication increases in school, at work, at home, or in the community. This can result in the following problems:

Expressive language is poorly organized when the person...
- ☐ Rambles in conversation or written work
- ☐ Interrupts with irrelevant ideas
- ☐ Gives minimal responses to questions and is unable to fill in details or offer other supporting information
- ☐ Finds it hard to organize thoughts and say what is on one's mind.

Inability to maintain attention can result in a person having...
- ☐ Poor listening when teachers are lecturing or bosses are giving directions
- ☐ Difficulty staying with a task long enough to complete it
- ☐ Difficulty responding in conversations because of losing the topic.

Difficulty with abstract language skills can cause a person to...
- ☐ Take what is said literally and not understand puns, sarcasm, or humor
- ☐ Have problems learning new information if generalizing or reasoning skills are needed.

Decreased rate of processing can result in a person...
- ☐ Needing extra time to understand what others are saying
- ☐ Reading slowly
- ☐ Finding it hard to understand what is read
- ☐ Having difficulty keeping up with complex sentences or vocabulary.

When a person with a brain injury has difficulty with cognitive communication and language, it is harder to learn and apply what is learned in daily life.

Who can treat these problems?

It is important to seek help from professionals who specialize in the assessment and treatment of persons with communication disabilities. Audiologists can assess hearing. Speech-language pathologists can assess specific communication problems, provide rehabilitation therapy and teach compensatory strategies.

These individuals may be licensed by their state and may possess a Certificate of Clinical Competence from the American Speech-Language-Hearing Association. They are employed in hospitals, clinics, universities, public schools, and private practice.

How Can Families and Friends Help?

Families, co-workers, teachers, and friends can play an important role in helping a person improve communication skills. They can help a person learn new compensatory strategies to reduce limitations.

Communication is a combination of speaking, listening, reading, writing, and gesturing. It does not have to be spoken. You can help by encouraging and accepting all forms of communication (written, gestured, or spoken) that help the person communicate.

Tips for improving communication...

✓ Be sure communication happens on a regular basis throughout the day.

✓ Use alternative means of communication such as pictures, reading, writing, gestures, and facial expressions if speaking does not seem to work.

✓ Respond to any and all attempts to communicate rather than focusing on verbal responses.

✓ Talk about familiar subjects and do not try to introduce new ideas without help.

✓ Consult with the speech-language pathologist before beginning practice of specific techniques such as rate of speech, breath control, or oral exercises.

✓ Be consistent in communication and establish what methods for communication will be used and be sure everyone uses the same techniques. (For example, if pointing to pictures is the method, no one should be requesting writing or verbal expression.)

✓ Keep conversation simple and direct, but at the correct age level of each family member.

✓ Ask questions and expect to be involved in the rehabilitation process and learn the compensatory strategies that are being taught.

Tips for monitoring yourself...

✓ Did this person understand what I said?

✓ Did I speak slowly enough?

✓ Did I give clear, step by step directions?

✓ Did I use puns or humor that was not understood?

✓ Can I help the person understand better by using pictures or writing the steps of what to do?

✓ Am I distracting this person with too many gestures, too loud a voice, or too many pauses in my speaking?

✓ Is the environment too loud, congested, bright, or confusing?

✓ Can I simplify this by speaking in shorter, clearer sentences?

✓ Can I give a more organized explanation of what I expect to be done?

✓ Who else can help?

Tips for what to do if you suspect there is a communication problem...

✓ Write down examples of the types of communication that concern you.

✓ Consider problems the environment might be causing.

✓ Analyze the communication manner and style of others and consider what changes could be made.

✓ Contact the medical professional you trust the most (regardless of professional discipline). Explain your observations and concerns and ask for a referral for a cognitive-communication evaluation by a speech-language pathologist.

✓ Expect the person with a brain injury and/or a family member to be included as a full team member in analyzing the communication problem and proposing solutions.

✓ Recognize that some expectations for improvement may be unrealistic and be prepared for using compensatory strategies rather than expecting full recovery.

✓ Ask to participate in setting goals and determining outcomes of treatment.

✓ Be sure treatment is directed toward improving the individual's ability to communicate well in home, school, work, or community activities.

✓ Learn to advocate that communication skills be considered when difficulty in school, work, or home begins.

Resource
The American Speech-Language and Hearing
Association
10801 Rockville Pike, Rockville, MD, 20852
www.asha.org Tel: 800-638-8255

Myths and Facts

About Behavior after Brain Injury
Written by: Harvey E. Jacobs, Ph.D.

✓ corrects common misunderstandings
✓ explains changes in behavior
✓ shows how to react positively

Understanding Behavior
What will he be like? Will she act differently now?

These are frequent questions of families. Over time, it is the changes in a person's social skills and behavior that usually concern families most. These changes in how the person acts can be more difficult to adjust to and manage than the initial medical and physical effects of a brain injury.

Not everybody's behavior will be affected or change the same way after a brain injury. Difficulties with behavior do not occur only for people with brain injury. For example, children and other family members may become upset or feel lost due to changes in routines, responsibilities and household resources. Their behavior may change as a result.

Here are some basic myths and facts about behavior after brain injury. Please use this information as a beginning guide and seek professional help, as needed, for your situation.

Myth...Brain injury causes behavior problems.
Fact... A person may act or behave differently because of changes in the brain after an injury or in reaction to how life has changed because of the injury.

A brain injury does not cause behavior problems by itself. But it may change how a person sees, hears, touches, smells, or otherwise senses what is happening or going on each day. It can change how a person remembers or understands information. It can change how a person responds or reacts to a situation.

Difficulties talking or communicating can also be frustrating. Emotional changes can be caused by damage to the brain or due to personal reactions of becoming disabled. Other changes can come from lost opportunities, such as not seeing old friends, not being able to go to work, losing freedom, or having less personal control.

When any of these changes cause problems, they are sometimes considered "behavior problems". But not all changes are a problem. It is important to remember that a brain injury itself does not cause a behavior problem, but it may set the stage for problems to occur.

Myth...He acts that way to get attention.
Fact... All people act in different ways to get attention.

Most people seek attention for their good deeds (positive attention) rather than for their misbehavior (negative attention). When people annoy others, it is usually because they don't know how to get attention in a more positive manner. They simply don't know what to do, are frustrated, cannot explain the problem, forgot what just happened, or past attempts at seeking positive attention failed.

Remember, the squeaky wheel gets the grease! When negative attention seeking occurs, such as arguing, refusing to do things, purposely throwing things or yelling, sit down with the person at a neutral time to discuss the situation. Find out what the person wants. Identify ways that everybody can work together, or at least come to a compromise. This will solve most situations. Understand how you, others, or the setting is contributing to the problem.

Myth...Punishing the person for the behavior will change it.
Fact... Punishing a person never works. Punishing a behavior may work temporarily, but there are much better approaches.

Punishment may briefly stop a behavior, but it rarely solves the problem. Many punishers cause negative emotional reactions that are stronger than the problem behavior. For example, always telling a person that something is being done the wrong way may cause the person to avoid you. This does little to improve personal relationships.

More effective and long-lasting approaches require understanding why the behavior occurs and helping the person find worthwhile alternatives. Sometimes the problem may be about motivation, sometimes about significant distress, and sometimes because the person doesn't know what else to do. Remember, this is about the individual, not you. Ignoring undesirable behavior, when it is not dangerous to do so, and paying attention to more desirable behavior, is a process known as differential reinforcement. It can be highly effective. But first, sit down and talk with the person to understand what is going on.

Myth...Anger means the person is out of control and is dangerous.
Fact... Anger occurs for many reasons.

At its most extreme levels, anger can indicate that a person is dangerously out of control. When this happens, make sure that everybody in the situation is safe until the immediate episode has ended. Seek outside help if necessary.

Anger can occur for many different reasons. A person may act angry because of frustration, problems communicating, feeling out of control, or not knowing what to do. Reassuring support once the person has calmed down can be very effective. Calmly find out what the person is trying to do and help find a successful solution. You may have to repeat this step often if the person has difficulty with memory or impulse control.

Damage within the emotional centers of the brain can cause the person to over-react, despite the person's efforts to remain calm. This requires help from physicians who may be able to prescribe medication. Psychologists and other professionals can assess contributing factors to the person's anger.

In other cases, anger may be a means of manipulation by the person to control others. This is often a sign of poor communication between parties. A counselor with training in the behavioral aspects of brain injury or a behavioral mediator may help.

Myth...Changes in behavior after brain injury are a sign of mental illness.
Fact... Behavior can change for many reasons, but it is usually not because of mental illness.

Changes in the way a person senses and experiences the world can change behavior, as can the changes in daily life. Many people feel depressed, anxious and have other emotional reactions to having a brain injury. These are realistic and understandable reactions to a devastating situation.

Problems develop when these reactions continue and interfere with self-care, relationships, adaptive skills, school, work and other areas of daily functioning. When this happens, assistance may be needed to help the person with the brain injury adapt - as well as help for the people living with or caring for the person. In such cases, it is best to seek help from a professional with experience in brain injury. A general health practitioner may not understand the special issues of life after brain injury and standard psychiatric approaches are not often effective.

Myth...Doing nothing, staying home and watching TV is a sign of laziness.
Fact... There are many reasons why a person will park in front of the TV.

Some people have difficulty with initiation and literally cannot get started, even when they want to –their get up and go has gotten up and went! They need help getting started and can often follow through when guided through the first few steps.

Some people may be depressed or socially withdraw due to poor self-esteem or despair. They may need encouragement to understand that others still value them – that they are not damaged goods.

Sometimes people have trouble trying different things, or adapting to new situations. Again, they may need encouragement and to be patiently led rather than pushed into new opportunities.

Most often, couch potatoism occurs due to lack of opportunities or inadequate transportation. Opportunities can end when past activities such as school, work, and social groups are no longer available. It's difficult to find engaging new opportunities and interesting people when the focus is on the disability. Focus on the person's interests and abilities instead. Try to re-engage the individual in the future rather than the past.

Myth...Avoidance is the safest approach when a person's behavior is unpredictable.

Fact... Unpredictable behavior usually indicates a problem that requires attention.

Behavior is generally predictable. Sometimes we just don't understand what causes the situation. This is why it is so important to involve the individual with the *problem* in evaluating and trying to solve the problem situation. Often there is a problem or difficulty communicating with other people. The situation itself can also contribute to the problem, especially if the person has trouble understanding or remembering important cues. Medication and health issues can affect behavior. Some individuals may be more vulnerable to their effects after a brain injury.

The key is to respectfully address the issue in a supportive and non-shaming manner. The goal is to improve life for everybody. Avoiding or sticking your head in the sand will do little to solve the problem.

Myth...Telling someone not to do something will only make things worse.

Fact... Helping someone be successful is a better approach.

Telling anybody what *not to do* without giving them an idea of *how to be successful* is a problem, whether or not they have a brain injury. There are situations where the individual or others are in danger where the only possible approach may be telling the person not to do something. However, a more successful solution is to find out what the person is trying to accomplish. Help the person decide what can be done to be successful in the situation. Help the person understand why the present approach may not be working or is in the best interests of others.

Myth...A person's behavior can be fixed if you just know what to do.

Fact... The behavior is not "broken" and people are not robots!

People and situations are constantly changing. Behavior represents how a person deals with daily life and responds to change. People age, jobs and financial situations change, other people enter and leave our lives, our health changes, and so on. *Fixing* a problem without understanding the dynamic nature of behavior is rarely successful. As soon as the situation changes, the problem will reappear. *Fixing* a problem without involving the primary person in the situation will also fail if the person does not have a say in the quality and direction of their life.

Behavior change is truly a process of behavior management. This begins with the primary person and the *positive* goals that the person is trying to accomplish. Once successful, it is then important to focus on how to sustain these goals and successes through the twists and turns of daily life.

Myth...With the right medication, the unwanted behavior will go away.

Fact... Medication is a tool, not an answer.

There is an unfortunate history of overmedication to subdue people who are acting out. Sometimes medication is used to sedate a person during early phases of rehabilitation to treat the injuries or because medical equipment or monitors require the person be quiet. Medication is also often used during this time when the person has an extreme level of confusion. However, this is not a successful long-term strategy. Many people become more agitated as the medication wears off. There can also be increased confusion from medication side effects.

Medication is best used to help improve daily functioning, rather than to suppress behavior. Some medications can improve alertness, arousal, attention and mood. There are medications used to reduce spasticity and improve movement disorders. However, most medications were developed for treating other conditions. Because each brain injury is unique, it is important to work with a physician experienced in treating people with brain injury to find the best available medication and dose. Beware that often there may not be medication to produce the desired effects.

Finally, medication alone is rarely the answer. Successful outcomes are best realized when medication is used with other daily therapies and supports to promote personal success.

Myth...People develop difficult personalities following a brain injury.

Fact... Notable personality traits may become more obvious following a brain injury, but are not always difficult!

Family members sometimes report that the person's personality traits become more obvious following a brain injury. Sometimes a person may become more stubborn, more withdrawn, or more emotional. Other people may show greater resolve, more focus, or more determination. This will obviously vary with the person and the situation. These changes are sometimes due to changes in awareness, impulse control, initiation, or agitation that may follow a brain injury. However, these changes can just as easily be due to a person trying to use the most familiar traits to address a challenging situation. It is important to work and relate with the person as an individual now, rather than how you would like the person to be.

Conclusion

Behavior changes after a brain injury for many reasons including:

- actual damage from the injury

- changes in cognition and communication

- psychological reaction to injury and disability; and

- social changes in a person's roles, relationships, resources and personal control.

Understanding these changes can prevent the start of problem behaviors. However, life following brain injury is complex. Problems, difficulties and challenges can occur for anybody who is involved. Begin by addressing these issues calmly and respectfully. Involve *all* parties in the process. Seek positive solutions and outcomes. Seek help from qualified and experienced professionals when problems continue. By focusing on positive methods of success, you can minimize the distress of failure.

References

Jacobs, H.E. (1993). *Behavior Analysis and Brain Injury Rehabilitation: People, Principles and Programs.* Gaithersburg, MD: Aspen Publishing Co.

McMorrow, M.J. (2003). *Getting Ready to Help: A Primer on Interacting in Human Service.* Baltimore, MD: Brookes Publishing Company.

Wood,R.L.(2001). McMillan-Wolfson (Ed.s) *Neurobehavioural Disability and Social Handicap Following Traumatic Brain Injury (Brain Damage, Behaviour and Cognition).* London, England: Taylor Francis Group.

Minding Behavior
Behavioral Challenges in Adults after Brain Injury
Written by: Harvey E. Jacobs, Ph.D.

✓ explains why behavior is functional
✓ gives positive approaches
✓ describes how to evaluate behavior

Introduction

Many people talk about "behavior problems" after brain injury. Sometimes the person with the brain injury complains of feeling anxious, depressed, or frustrated. Often somebody else recognizes the problem. For example, a wife feels that her husband is more moody than before his injury. A supervisor notes that a worker no longer follows through on orders. Friends learn that they can't disagree with Ralph anymore because he loses his temper.

Problems often occur when a person is not aware of or has trouble monitoring behavior. For example, the person may take over a conversation, continue telling jokes that others find offensive, or mistake an innocent gaze as an invitation for flirtation. The kitchen may be a mess after a "cooking episode" because the person got frustrated that the cake did not rise, went to pieces when an ingredient wasn't on hand, or did not clean up afterwards being "unaware" of the mess.

It is too easy to simply blame the brain injury. There are many other factors to consider, including:

- what the person was like before the brain injury
- current skills and abilities
- what is now expected of the person
- the daily living environment
- resources and supports in the person's life
- behavior of other people, and
- normal changes over the lifespan.

Brain injury may change a person's life, but it should never define a person's life!

What is Behavior?

Consider behavior as a journey rather than a destination. Too many people see behavior as some solely fixable thing that is the primary cause of other problems, e.g. "Why can't you fix Alex's anger!" It is important to think of behavior as a fluid and dynamic process of a person interacting with the environment. The resulting "products" that we see are behavior.

People and environments are very complex. Many different things affect each. People are influenced by:

- how they feel
- medications
- medical, physical and neurological status
- emotions
- life experiences
- skills and abilities
- faith; and
- many other variables

The demands of the environment affect how we react. Is this a new or unfamiliar setting? What cues and guides, *that are meaningful to us,* are present in the situation? Are we being expected to do something we are comfortable with or something different? What is at stake for us and for others? What makes us feel happy, sad, angry, fearful, confused, or numb in the situation? What do other people expect of us? Who are the other people? *This interaction of the person and the environment produces behavior.*

Behavior May Be Dysfunctional, But Never Disordered!

Behavior is not magical – there is always a reason for it. Difficulties develop when the skills and abilities of the individual do not match the demands of the situation. This may happen because the person does not have the skills or capability, or because others do not understand or realize this. For example, an injured worker returns to the "same old job" but with new limitations that neither the person nor the employer understands. The person fails or "causes" other people to fail, becomes upset or "makes" other people upset, or acts in some way that is not helpful to anyone.

Our "behavioral functionality," or competency, is determined by how we respond in a given situation. Our behavior is considered *functional or competent* when we react in *customary and acceptable* ways. Our behavior may be considered *dysfunctional or incompetent*, when we react in *uncustomary or unacceptable* ways.

Many behavioral challenges occur when we face a new situation. We often try to rely on past experiences and respond as in a previous "almost similar" situation. It's important to understand how a situation can be new.

- *First, the environment or other people can be new.*

  Examples are moving to a new city and figuring out where to shop, starting a new job and learning how to operate new equipment, or establishing a new relationship and interacting with a new personality.

- *Second, the person and their abilities may have changed even though everything else is the same.*

  This often happens following brain injury. Changes in memory may mean you forget what used to come naturally; changes in physical ability can affect strength, endurance, or other aspects of work that used to be easy; changes in emotional lability can affect how you respond to a situation.

- *Third, it's usually a combination of these that change as roles, responsibilities, expectations, and abilities change for <u>everyone</u> involved. With these changes come changes in everybody's behavior!*

We can usually find perfectly good reasons why the "problem" behavior occurred, even if there is little that we can do about the situation. While the behavior may be dysfunctional, it is not disordered. There is always at least one reason why it occurred.

Judging and Evaluating Behavior

Dysfunctional behavior becomes an even bigger challenge when others react dysfunctionally. It's difficult to remain calm when someone physically threatens you, not to feel a loss when your continuing offers of intimacy are not reciprocated, or to hold your tongue when being verbally berated.

One of the biggest challenges is to maintain perspective and not sacrifice the individual because of the behavior. It's too easy to judge the person, rather than evaluate the specific behavior. We naturally decide not to be involved with this "bad person" for our safety. We may be uncomfortable around someone whose behavior is never predictable. We may judge this person as weird and may attribute it to bad genes, the brain injury, or some other unchangeable condition. Having made this judgment, we begin to always view this person this way. We are judging – coming to conclusions based on our personal reactions and biases.

Evaluating behavior requires looking at the big picture and putting aside emotions to objectively consider many factors:

- *"Thee before me"*

  Understand why someone engages in the behavior before reacting. Walk a mile in the person's shoes!

- *"State, then trait"*

  Identify the environment and context in which the behavior occurs. Understand how the person is likely to respond based on past experiences and personality. Given what you know about this person, are you surprised or assured by what happened?

- *"Intensity and propensity"*

  Identify the intensity of the behavior as well as its propensity (frequency). Sometimes a person gets "marked" because of one episode that colors everything else. In extreme examples, this may be an appropriate consideration (e.g., extreme violence), but often it's not. A behavior with a minor negative effect may occur so frequently that its level of annoyance far exceeds its true problematic status.

- *"Good, Gooder, Goodest"*

  The quality of a behavior may pose a challenge. A person may not complete a task to some expected level of performance. There can also be situations where the person spends too much time doing a better job than needed in one area, to the neglect of other priorities. Behavioral competency is as much about *when to do* something, as *how well* to do it.

So, What Are You Going to Do?

Successful behavior change requires a commitment by everyone. Too many people presume that behavioral interventions involve getting people to start or stop something they don't want to. This approach is rarely effective and often counterproductive.

Behavior change is most effective when all parties are involved. The person identified as having "the problem" *must* be involved from the start. This is more than an issue of dignity and respect – it is also common sense. Most "behavior problems" are really problems of communication and resolve as people understand reciprocal needs and expectations. When communication alone can't resolve the problem, it can set the venue for further progress.

People can choose to participate or not. Sometimes an outside party is needed to help mediate the situation. However, interventions will fail if the principals do not have a say in its direction and a stake in its results.

There has to be a good reason for *all* parties to change behavior. Other people sometimes have a vested interest in continuing the problem. For example, if the person becomes more independent, then other people may also need to change. Change can be uncomfortable for anybody.

The good news is that most people want to make the change – *if they think it is for the better.* This requires focusing on positive goals - what each person has to gain, rather than what is wrong and needs to be removed.

Behavior Has a Purpose

Successful behavior change involves finding more acceptable, productive, and functional ways for the person to achieve the goal and for others to support this change.

Programs designed to stop "bad behavior" rarely offer this focus and generally fail. These types of programs tell you what not to do, but not how to get what you want or need. For example, weight reduction programs that principally focus on not eating generally fail. Too often we assume that simply removing the "bad" behavior makes "good" behaviors magically appear. A more successful approach involves teaching people how to enjoy more healthy foods.

Knowing Where You Are Going

Behavioral interventions are not simply designing consequences to behavior. Many approaches can be used once positive goals and resources are identified. Do your homework ahead of time and make sure that everybody agrees on the goals – the more specific, the better. This also helps prevent multiple or hidden agendas.

Resources include time, people, access to services, funding, and other supports. Goals may need to change or be modified if the resources don't match. Too many people fail because they don't consider what they truly need to meet their goals. It is better to successfully modify your overall goal into several steps than to run out of gas midstream.

Effective behavior change requires resources and supports over time. Sometimes these come from the same resources and supports that sustain the problem situation by reallocating these resources in a more productive manner. Other times additional resources are needed. Everybody must have a stake in the entire process.

Knowing When You Get There

It's important to frequently measure your progress towards desired goals so you can make any needed mid-course corrections to stay on track. Remember that you are dealing with dynamic events that are likely to change. Your focus is on *outcome*.

Methods of measurement can be very simple *if* the behavioral goals are clearly understood. For example:

- Work quality of the employee on the job
- Nights you and your mate end up falling asleep snuggling in the same bed compared to someone ending up on the couch
- School grades and test results
- Percentage of conversations that are on positive rather than complaining topics
- Hours per day that the caregiver is able to be alone.

Conclusion

Behavior is a reflection of our lives. It is a dynamic entity under constant change. Focusing on the opportunities over the difficulties, and understanding all parties who are involved in a "behavioral problem" allows us to re-establish the regard, respect and dignity that are so vital to personal commerce.

Reference

Jacobs, H.E. (1993). *Behavior Analysis Guidelines and Brain Injury Rehabilitation: People, Principles and Programs.* Gaithersburg, MD: Aspen.

Ylvisaker, M and Feeney, T.J. (1998). *Collaborative Brain Injury Intervention: Positive everyday routines.* San Diego, CA: Singular Publishing Group.

Behavior at Home
Managing Challenges in Adults after Brain Injury
Written by: Carolyn Rocchio & Harvey E. Jacobs, Ph.D.

✓ develop successful strategies
✓ correct misinformation about behavior

Educating the Family

Family members usually absorb only a portion of the information they receive while a member is in the hospital or rehabilitation program. The entire experience is overwhelming for most people. Some report that there is just too much information to digest in too short a period of time. Others report that they receive little or no information about brain injury. Few people understand the difference between illness and disability during the early stages of brain injury recovery. Many expect that the physician and rehabilitation specialists will "cure" or "fix" the problem before the person is discharged. This is not possible and may set up a family for many future difficulties.

Example: Frank offers to empty the dishwasher after dinner but is interrupted by a ringing telephone. After answering the telephone, he fails to return and complete the chore. His wife then yells at him for not finishing, words are exchanged, and the whole scene quickly gets out of hand.

The outcome might have been very different had Frank and his wife understood that he now has problems with concentration and follow-through, but benefits from external cueing. In this situation Frank would likely have completed the job and the couple could have enjoyed each other's company for the night if his wife knew to say, "Thank you for answering the telephone. I hope you can finish putting away the dishes without more interruptions."

Educating families is an involved process that takes time. Not all problems are readily apparent following a brain injury. It is important that family members understand not only what abilities have been damaged following a brain injury, but also what abilities are intact or preserved.

Cognitive and Behavioral Changes

These are the changes after a brain injury that are often more difficult for families to adapt to than the physical challenges. This holds true whether the person with a brain injury is a spouse, parent, sibling or child. It is easy for most people to understand how a physical disability can affect a person's life because the changes are often visible. It is often obvious why a person has difficulty when an arm or leg is missing or damaged.

Changes in how a person acts or thinks after a brain injury usually do not have such obvious markers. Damage within the brain cannot be seen so easily. It's not unusual to hear a family member say, "I just don't understand why she gets so angry now and doesn't take responsibility for anything." The family member's frustration or irritation may be confusing to the person with the brain injury. This can be stressful and frustrating for everyone. These changes can pose the greatest challenge to a person's independence and a productive life at home and in the community.

Most people with brain injury go directly home from the hospital. A few are admitted to inpatient rehabilitation programs for short periods before returning home. It is difficult to educate and prepare families during this brief time. As a result, families are rarely prepared to understand, much less supervise, a family member with cognitive and behavioral challenges. Yet, with proper education, guidance and direction, most families and people with brain injury can avoid or minimize the negative long-term effects of these challenges.

Work Toward Success

The challenges of life with brain injury can affect all family members. Services work best when they focus on promoting everybody's success. Structure, consistency, concreteness, patience and everybody's participation are critical for success. Here are some common beliefs about managing challenging behaviors at home and in the community with tips on strategies for success.

Belief #1: *Behavior programs are principally designed to stop unwanted and dangerous behaviors.*

False - Successful behavioral programs focus on helping people be more productive, engaged and involved in their daily lives according to their interests, responsibilities and abilities. Programs principally designed to stop "bad behavior" are rarely successful. They can actually increase rather than improve the problem over time.

Tips on strategies for success…
✓ Focus on abilities over disabilities.
✓ Include the person with a brain injury in all program planning from the beginning.
✓ Involve all family members and caregivers.
✓ Identify problems and opportunities early and start to work on them as soon as possible.

Belief #2: *Successful behavior management programs developed in rehabilitation settings will automatically work at home and in the community.*

False - Techniques practiced in rehabilitation will not automatically work at home or in the community. The settings and people involved are different. But well designed behavior programs can usually be adapted to home and community.

Tips on strategies for success…
✓ Identify major differences in a person's daily routine at home compared to the rehabilitation setting.
✓ Make sure that the person with the brain injury and family members are involved in developing strategies that are practical for them.
✓ Identify who will be participating and provide them with very specific training.
✓ Review approaches on a regular basis to see if they are working and revise as needed.

Belief #3: *Family members are more easily manipulated and cannot manage home behavioral programs.*

False - Although a certain amount of manipulation exists in any close relationship, most family members can learn to be effective agents for behavior change and support.

Tips on strategies for success…
✓ Recognize the strengths and limits of each family member or caregiver.
✓ Identify what help and support families will need to consistently and successfully use developed programs and strategies.
✓ Train and educate families about the individual's difficulties and abilities.
✓ Involve the person with the brain injury in program development to improve chances for continuing success.
✓ Give the person control and choices in areas where he/she can responsibly and safely exercise control.

Belief #4: *One person in the family should be responsible for managing the behavioral program.*

True - One individual should be the identified "manager" to coordinate the behavioral program, but everyone needs to be involved.

Tips on strategies for success…
✓ Have the manager help everybody who lives in the household, especially the person with the brain injury, become familiar with program strategies.
✓ Make sure that everyone consistently follows the programming.
✓ Set up a structure for the day or activity that can be consistently followed, yet is flexible enough to allow for unexpected events.
✓ Maintain a collaborative role with all parties at all times, continually assuring that everybody understands the program's purpose and procedures, and has the support they need to participate.

Belief #5: *Structured and supervised settings are impossible to manage when family members must work and maintain their schedules.*

False - Structuring and scheduling are even more critical to help this household function in the least disruptive manner.

Tips on strategies for success…
✓ Organize the activities of family members to ensure that a responsible person is available in the house at all times, or as often as possible.
✓ Post a written schedule that everybody can follow in case plans change, or if someone has to be contacted.
✓ Have an alternative plan for self-management to help the person with the brain injury meet any immediate needs when no one is available.

Belief #6: *My child or spouse has always been a gentle person. Although he has very aggressive behavior now, I know that he will not strike me.*

False - It is very important to understand the situation when such types of behavior occur. Some people may strike out, often at those with whom they are closest. Some will vent their frustrations toward others.

Tips on strategies for success...
✓ Have a method for stopping or redirecting behavior before it results in serious consequences. This may be a cue to help the person stop and consider if he/she is confused or needs other help. The cue may distract the person, or reduce immediate stress and demands.
✓ Protect the individual's safety as well as your own if the behavior continues.
✓ Have a plan to get outside help fast in cases of severe behavioral problems, severe aggression or self-injury. Make sure the person cannot harm him/herself.
✓ Call for professional help, including paramedics or 911 when facing an emergency. Everybody's safety is imperative in such situations.
✓ Get professional help to assess and develop a plan to address such situations in the future.

Belief #7: *My family member acts unfeeling and seems uncaring when others are ill or in need of help.*

True and False - Some people with brain injury show a loss of empathy and inability to relate to others. This can be due to changes in awareness of situations or how they relate to others. It can be caused by changes in emotional reactions, depression, or other factors. Some people feel empathy but can no longer express it. Understanding the cause of this lack of empathy may help both of you to relate better and understand one another.

Tips on strategies for success...
✓ Discuss the issue calmly and non-judgmentally. Seek to identify if the person is unaware of the situation, is depressed, doesn't care, or what else is going on.
✓ Develop strategies to let the person know when it is really important to respond to a situation. You may have to use cues or reminders to get the person involved.
✓ Understand your own reactions when the person does not respond to your needs. You may be more upset about the situation than the other person is. You may need to find support from others. Understand how this may positively or negatively affect your relationship with your family member.

Belief #8: *The use of medications to manage behavior should be a last resort.*

False - Effective use of appropriate medications that help improve awareness, attention, understanding, mood, energy or self-control should always be considered. Problems develop when medications are primarily used to suppress unwanted behaviors, or when they are used without understanding the side effects on a person's productive skills. Medications may have different and often paradoxical effects on a person following a brain injury than for people without brain injury. This even includes "simple" medications such as pain relievers, decongestants, etc.

Tips on strategies for success...
✓ Work with a physician who has experience prescribing medications for people with brain injury.
✓ Make sure the focus of medication management is to help a person succeed in daily activities.
✓ Understand that because brain injury can change the effects of medication, different medications or dosages may have to be tried to reach desired effects.

Belief #9: *A gradual or severe change in behavior can indicate the development of a psychosis, mental illness or dementia.*

True and False - These changes can occur for many reasons such as illness, other disease processes, improper nutrition, medication side effects, personal or family history, etc. It is not always the brain injury or a psychiatric condition.

Tips on strategies for success...
✓ Have a physician experienced in working with people with behavioral challenges following brain injury evaluate and assess such changes.
✓ Make sure other issues that may be contributing to the behavior are considered.

Belief #10: *I can't do anything about the person running away or wandering from the house.*

False - People may leave the house for many reasons including being bored, wanting to go somewhere to do something, or easily getting lost (even after just walking out the door) and being unable to find the way home. Locking people in the house rarely works and upsets everybody.

Tips on strategies for success...
✓ Make sure that the person has enough structured interests and activities within and outside the home to reduce wandering.

✓ Consider an alarm on doors and windows to cue you when the person leaves the house.

✓ If such problems occur frequently, let local police and other authorities know and teach them how to respond to the person and get them back home.

✓ Encourage the person to wear a Medic Alert, a regular ID bracelet or other form of identification to be easily recognized and returned home.

Conclusion

Changes in behavior and cognition may be some of the most enduring and frustrating challenges for people with brain injuries and their families. Identifying the personal challenges and helping people find successful routes in daily living through supportive programming can reduce stress and burden for everybody. Planning and developing programs begin by involving the person with a brain injury. Different programs will work in different settings and for different people. Most family members can learn how to address many of these issues. It is also important to consider the guidance and direction of experienced professionals.

Behavior Programs and Behavior Problems

Promote Success and Avoid Failure

Written by: Harvey E. Jacobs, Ph.D.

✓ understand least restrictive programming
✓ minimize or prevent seclusion and restraint
✓ identify positive and proactive services

Challenges of Behavior after Brain Injury

Some people have very challenging and dangerous behaviors after brain injury. They may hurt or threaten others, damage property, try to hurt themselves, or run away. These problems often can be resolved with positive behavioral programming, counseling, education, medication and/or other treatment.

Successful programming helps individuals develop better social skills, find things of interest to do, learn better ways to communicate, manage frustration, return to school or work, and live in the community. Difficult behaviors usually fade away when opportunities are developed that are valued and important for the individual.

Example - Carl was expelled from school for being aggressive and not completing his work. Classes were one hour long, but Carl could only concentrate for five minutes at a time. He had problems understanding what people said. His new school broke tasks into five-minute sections and gave him written rather than spoken directions. Carl loved learning and succeeded with these changes.

Example – Stacey rarely got dressed, started fights and disrupted everybody's lives. She was diagnosed with borderline personality disorder. She was smart, bored, and didn't care much for people, but she loved animals. All these problems vanished when she started volunteering at a local animal shelter. She couldn't wait to get up each day for work or tell others about her job at the end of the day.

Behavior Programs Can Cause Behavior Problems

Well-designed behavioral programs help people succeed; poorly designed programs do not. An individual who has "problem behavior" may be seen as a "problem person" in some programs. The treatment may not fit the problem unless the person and situation are fully understood. It may even make the problem worse. Behavior that is identified as a problem may be a reflection of other more serious issues.

Example - Mack was given "emergency medication" and restricted to his room after assaulting his physical therapist. He was discharged to a psychiatric hospital. No one knew he was a former prisoner of war who had been tied to a chair for days at a time. He had flashbacks when the therapist put a lap belt on him. He was simply scared. With assurance, he would have cooperated with staff.

Example - Joy refused her daily care and began urinating on the furniture. It was "clear" that she had oppositional-defiant behavior. A program was started to physically force her to do things and clean the room after an accident. Three months later, staff realized that the shunt in her brain was clogged and building up fluid. The "problem" went away, but not her emotional trauma from the episode.

Challenging behavior can occur for many reasons. Even small issues can cause big reactions when programming is inconsistent or insensitive to a person's needs. Programs with inadequate treatment environments, inexperienced or insufficient staff, inadequate resources, and improper clinical focus can produce far more behavioral problems than "problem patients." Unfortunately, it is the patients who often suffer the most.

It is very important for treatment to fit the need, but it is even more important that the need be properly understood to select the proper treatment. Otherwise, people face ineffective or possibly harmful procedures that can cause more problems than they solve.

Least Restrictive Treatment

Some behaviors are so severe or dangerous that they require more intensive and restrictive approaches to reduce their occurrence. Treatment is usually ranked from the least to most restrictive according to the behavior being addressed and the procedure being used.

Least restrictive – These are procedures that interfere the least with a person's abilities to follow a daily schedule and continue regular activities.

More restrictive - The more a treatment procedure or program interferes with a person's daily life, the more restrictive it is.

Example - A person who voluntarily leaves a room to calm down when becoming upset is using a procedure called time-out. This is less restrictive than forcibly removing and placing a person alone in a room until staff gives permission to leave (a procedure called seclusion). Time-out is not always a less restrictive procedure. It depends on the specific treatment goals and behaviors. For example, rewarding a person for desired behavior is a less restrictive procedure than using time out when teaching social skills.

Note - It's not always possible to use the least restrictive procedure, especially if it is unlikely to work or the person is in immediate danger. For example, ignoring an outburst when a person is at immediate risk of hurting others could be harmful.

Understanding seclusion and restraint

Highly restrictive procedures, such as seclusion and restraint, may be needed when behavior is so dangerous that it places the individual or others in severe harm and no other procedure will work. In most cases, there is a better alternative. Seclusion and restraint are emergency procedures; they are not effective treatment for challenging behavior.

People with especially challenging or dangerous behaviors are the most vulnerable to seclusion and restraint. When a program is unable to adapt to an individual's special needs, behavior may deteriorate and lead to a very unsafe or dangerous situation. This may result in the use of seclusion, restraint or other highly restrictive procedures. Unfortunately, many patients and staff are injured and some die from the misuse of such procedures each year.

Any treatment program that principally focuses on reducing problem behaviors is unacceptable. Programs that follow best practices focus on positive goals, increased abilities and personal self-direction. They rarely have to use more restrictive procedures and consider them temporary measures when necessary.

Federal and state guidelines on seclusion and restraint vary, but there are basic guidelines.

Seclusion - isolates a person from others and physically prevents the person from leaving a confined area. It includes…

- placing a person alone in a locked room
- putting a person in solitary confinement
- preventing a person from leaving a room by blocking the doorway, etc.

Restraint - This involves any means by which others restrict movement or access to a person's body that is against a person's will It includes…

- having other people hold a person
- restricting movement through straps, belts, helmets, or other mechanical means
- using medications principally to subdue a person's actions (chemical restraint)

Medical restraints are special exceptions that protect a person from the consequences of a medical condition. Examples are wearing a helmet to protect the head during seizures or using a lap belt to protect a person from falling out of a wheel chair. A physician must authorize and review the use of these restraints. They must be designed so that the person or guardian can independently decide when to use and remove them.

Using seclusion and restraint

Seclusion and restraint are generally not legal in community-based programs such as group homes, day programs and nursing homes, but may still occur. These procedures may be allowed in hospitals and other special settings depending on their clinical license. It varies among states.

Seclusion and restraint are emergency procedures. The treatment team must review the individual's program within 24 hours whenever seclusion and restraint are used to determine why the problem occurred. The team must also modify the individual's program to prevent their use in the future.

Unfortunately, this becomes a paperwork exercise with some programs continuing these procedures. Some programs may still use seclusion and restraint, but call them something else such as emergency medication for chemical restraint, forced relaxation for seclusion, etc. Programs that regularly use seclusion and restraint may not have the clinical ability to address challenging behavior in a positive manner. They should be approached with extreme caution.

It is important for everyone involved to know their rights and responsibilities about restrictive procedures. Families and other advocates should stay involved and ask questions. They should require the program to inform them when restrictive procedures are being considered and each time they are used. A good place to learn more about individual rights and responsibilities is with each state's Office of Protection and Advocacy, or the Office of Human Rights. Phone numbers are located in the state government sections of the phone book. There are also many resources available through the internet.

Elements of Effective Behavior Programs

Positive key factors in programs for people with challenging behaviors include …

- Involvement of the individual, family, friends and other stakeholders as key team members from the beginning
- Staff that is well-trained, stable and experienced in brain injury
- Low turnover in direct care and clinical staff
- Programs and staff with the time and resources required for success
- Focus on a person's abilities rather than disabilities
- Routine evaluation of all factors affecting behavior
- Use of best practices for behavior analysis
- Routine use of least restrictive treatment
- Collection of daily data to determine program direction and needed changes
- Services in setting most relevant to the client
- Natural supports to maintain successful behavior change
- High regard of program by consumers, professionals and service agencies
- Acknowledgement of abilities and limitations - no program can do everything!

Finding a Program – what to look for and avoid

Few programs will meet all these criteria. Not every program works for everybody. Services vary by region. It's important to ask questions and talk with staff when looking for a program that can address specific behavior challenges for a person with a brain injury.

Tips for evaluating potential services…

✓ Be wary of intake evaluations that focus on how a person can fit within a program, rather than how a program will adapt for a person. Good programs adapt to the individual's needs, not the other way around.

✓ Ask for specific details and examples. Don't accept "lip service" or general explanations. People who know what they are doing can explain things in detail and are proud of their work.

✓ Inquire about credentials and experience of the staff. Beware of many staff with provisional rather than full licensure.

✓ Ask if administrators/top management staff have relevant clinical training and experience.

✓ Get an overall impression if staff appear competent and organized or overwhelmed.

✓ Observe how staff interact with individuals in the program.

✓ Avoid programs with frequent staff turnover, especially among direct care and clinical staff.

✓ Look at the physical design and organization of the program to determine if it promotes adaptive skills or mainly reacts to problem behaviors (for example, lots of locked doors, time out rooms, and restrictive procedures versus a wide range of activities and opportunities that meet the needs and interests of the people served).

✓ Find out how clients like the program when possible.

✓ Visit the program with a scheduled appointment.

✓ Drop in for an unexpected visit and see how staff and administration respond.

✓ Stay away from programs that can do everything!!!! They can't!

There is no perfect program. What works for one person may not work for another.

Keep Things Going Well

Finding the right program and keeping it focused are two different issues. It's important for families and other concerned parties to stay involved during the individual's treatment. Make sure that programs keep their promises, but even more importantly, that everyone else keeps theirs. This includes family members, case managers, funding sources and other involved parties. Poor communication is the biggest reason for treatment failure. Changes in personal commitment, emotional reserve, resources, and changes in program operations can affect results. Treatment is a dynamic process that involves constant communication and adaptation.

Conclusion

Finally, don't try to do it alone, especially when addressing highly challenging behavior. Understand that you are likely to be in crisis when seeking help and it is important to think clearly and strategically. This means thinking about long-term goals as well as the immediate need. Get help from professionals, support groups, advocates and consumers to locate and evaluate resources.

References

Jacobs, H.E. (1993). *Behavior Analysis Guidelines and Brain Injury Rehabilitation: People, Principles and Programs.* Gaithersburg, MD: Aspen Publishing Company.

McMorrow, M.J. (2005). *The Helping Exchange: P.E.A.R.L.* Wake Forest, NC: Lash and Associates Publishing/Training Inc.

Gross, G. (2003). *Restraint and Seclusion – Overview of Federal Laws and Policies.* Washington, D.C.: National Association of Protection and Advocacy Systems.

Changes in Self Awareness
After a Brain Injury
Written by: McKay Moore Sohlberg, Ph.D.

✓ understand sources and types of unawareness
✓ use strategies to lesson effects of unawareness

Why is Self Awareness Important?

Self awareness is the ability to view ourselves somewhat objectively. It is also the ability to see ourselves from the perspective of other people. It allows us to use feedback from others as we develop our personal identity. We rely on self awareness when we…

- interact socially with others
- decide what situations or information to share
- make judgments about ourselves, and
- act in ways that insure our personal safety.

Brain injury can impair the critical capacity for self awareness. This can result in many problems for the individual who has been injured as well as the family. Research has shown that impaired self awareness often limits or slows down recovery. Individuals may not follow therapy recommendations or participate in supportive efforts because they do not recognize that they have a problem. Several studies have shown that employment outcomes for people with impaired self awareness are lower than for people who don't experience this difficulty after brain injury.

The caregivers of people with brain injury who have poor self awareness also tend to report greater levels of stress. Caregivers may find themselves arguing with a person displaying unawareness when this person does not see or acknowledge the problem. This can be especially challenging when it involves personal safety or danger. Understanding the nature of unawareness and becoming familiar with some basic management strategies may help those who care for or treat people with awareness deficits.

Sources of Unawareness

"My husband does not seem to be unhappy about his condition, but he lacks insight about what he can and cannot do. He will ask when he is going back to work or suggest that he could help me drive the kids when it seems so obvious that he does not have the physical or cognitive abilities to do these activities. When I explain that he cannot drive or work because of his brain injury, he does not object. He just doesn't get how his impairments affect his ability to do daily tasks."

"When I remind my daughter to use her memory system she becomes extremely angry and yells at me that she doesn't need the book or any other type of help. She says she's totally fine now and that we just won't recognize that she's better."

Impairments in self awareness are complex. They can arise from many different causes. The particular responses of individuals with impaired self awareness may differ widely from one another. Consider how the following possible sources of impairments in self awareness may contribute to inaccurate self judgments by an individual with a brain injury.

Source 1: Direct injury to brain structures responsible for awareness

Certain parts of the brain provide information to a person about how he or she is functioning. For example, the frontal brain regions behind the forehead are generally thought to significantly contribute to a person's insight and judgment. In some cases, people may be able to describe changes in their abilities, but they do not appreciate how the changes affect their lives. For example, a person may acknowledge having a severe memory impairment and difficulty learning new information, but feel able to successfully complete rigorous college courses.

Sometimes damage to a particular area of the brain causes a very specific type of unawareness. For example, damage to specific locations in the right brain hemisphere can cause unawareness of a person's left sided paralysis.

Source 2: Direct injury to structures responsible for thinking processes

Brain damage that affects memory or problem solving may also contribute to unawareness. If a person cannot remember information or does not fully understand it, that information cannot be used effectively. For example, impaired reasoning may result in a lack of understanding about the demands of a task. The person may attempt an activity that is unsafe because the person cannot anticipate possible consequences. Problems with judgment or awareness can stem from cognitive impairments.

Source 3: Psychological denial

Denial is sometimes confused with unawareness. Denial occurs when a person knows that he or she may have difficulties, but suppresses this information. The person may soften or outright deny evidence that reveals limitations. This is a psychological issue rather than the direct result of a brain injury. Psychological denial is an emotional defense mechanism that can spare a person the pain of recognizing difficulties and losses. To some degree it is normal and, in some cases, can be functional if it is not too extreme.

Source 4: No opportunity to experience changes

Occasionally an individual simply has not had the opportunity to experience the changes brought on by a brain injury. A cognitive impairment does not hurt like a broken leg. A person may think he or she is fine until experience shows otherwise. For example, a person may think that he can still drive because he has not yet tried it. Lack of such awareness may be apparent in the initial months following an injury while the person is gradually returning to routine activities and experiencing changes.

Often, more than one source contributes to changes in self awareness. A person may have some denial of deficits in addition to diminished self awareness due to brain damage. Awareness is complex and may take many different forms. A person may appear to have awareness or *knowledge* about personal strengths and limitations but be unable to *apply* that knowledge and make appropriate judgments about capabilities. Different awareness profiles often require different responses.

What Helps Unawareness?

The primary reason to work on awareness is to help people make better decisions. It is critical that efforts to increase a person's understanding of his or her abilities and disabilities are done in a manner that preserves self esteem. A healthy sense of self is critical for recovery.

The two primary methods to address impaired self awareness are education and structured feedback. Both require an interpersonal bond between the person delivering information or feedback and the individual with impaired self awareness. It is also important to have an environment that helps the person learn about strengths and weaknesses while still maintaining hope.

Education

Educational approaches to improve self awareness often involve teaching a person about the effects of brain injury. Education may begin with general information and then move to individualized education about a person's situation. Researchers have described systematic educational procedures such as...

- reviewing and helping interpret people's medical records
- jointly reading articles or books
- viewing media materials on relevant topics, or
- assigning generative activities (e.g., designing a presentation for a group on a brain injury topic).

Education is particularly helpful for people who have not had an opportunity to experience changes. It also may be useful for people who have unawareness of specific types of deficits. For example, education may be used to instruct an individual that her brain injury makes it difficult for her to recognize that her arm is paralyzed. This may be the first step in teaching a person to compensate for a deficit. When providing education, it is important to deliver information in a way that recognizes and provides accommodations for any cognitive impairments (e.g., use of graphics or the construction of a brain injury education notebook that a person can refer to as needed.)

Feedback

One of the most common forms of intervention for improving self-awareness is giving feedback. Therapists may use direct feedback when they are working with clients in sessions. Alternatively feedback may be given on videotape samples.

Sometimes indirect feedback is more productive for individuals whose awareness issues stem primarily from psychological denial. Indirect feedback may take the form of allowing people to self monitor their improvement on tasks over time. For example, a person may keep a log of successes and challenges on a specific home or work task. Signs or evidence of improvement can help the client understand that earlier performance was impaired. It also helps the client see the gains that have been made over time and that future gains are still needed or possible.

The goal of feedback is to orient individuals to the aspects of their performance that they do not accurately perceive. It is very important in this process to balance feedback for problem areas with feedback for strengths.

Regardless of the approach used to help someone increase self awareness, the person in the role of therapist, coach or care provider needs to have a positive bond or connection with the individual. In order for a person to accept feedback, the person needs to feel that there is a partnership. The clinical term for this partnership is therapeutic alliance.

Communicating about Unawareness

It is helpful to remember that working on awareness is a *process*. There are few, if any, quick fixes. Unawareness represents a complex dynamic between emotional and cognitive functioning. Optimizing communication may improve opportunities to increase awareness.

Tips for therapists and caregivers…
✓ Try to align yourself with the individual and avoid power struggles.

No one likes to hear about personal shortcomings. Directly confronting or arguing about the presence of an impairment usually entrenches a person in the belief that there is no problem. This is particularly true for people with problems of denial. Try to find strengths and points of agreement and use encouraging language by positively restating difficulties and offering compromises.

Examples of positive restatements:
"I am impressed with your determination to be independent. I understand why you want to pursue this and your drive will help you get there. I'll try to not get in the way and only remind you about the big stuff."

"I don't want to work on things you don't need

help with or hold you back. So let's figure out what pieces of this are easy and which are more difficult."

Examples of compromise:
"Would you be willing to try the medication for a month and if it doesn't seem to be working after that we can relook at things?"

"Would you be more comfortable if the job coach sat in the back instead of right next to you?"

✓ Preserve self esteem

Make sure attempts to increase a person's awareness strike a balance between confrontation and support.

- Make lists of attributes that were not affected by the brain injury
- Focus on strengths
- Reinforce progress
- Avoid only giving attention to problems

Conclusion

Awareness deficits can be very frustrating for families, support people and individuals with brain injury. People who have limited awareness of the type, extent or impact of their impairments may resist using accommodations or may make poor choices. Some may fight helpful suggestions because they feel others are being critical about issues that, in their view, do not exist. Other times, people may feel that the "help" of others restricts their freedom and daily activities. Finally, the person who has problems of awareness may appear to simply not care. This can be especially frustrating for a person's partners, whether they are family members, friends or business associates.

Helping people have a realistic appraisal of their abilities and challenges can be a complex process. This applies to both people who experience disability following brain injury and the people around them. Above all, addressing challenges of awareness requires a positive rapport and careful communication among all parties.

References

Sherer, M. (2005). Rehabilitation of impaired awareness. In WM. High, AM. Sander, MA Struchen and KA Hart (eds) *Rehabilitation for Traumatic Brain Injury*. New York: Oxford University Press, 31-46.

Fleming, JM, Strong, J. & Ashton, R. (1996). Self-awareness of deficits in adults with traumatic brain injury: How best to measure? *Brain Injury* 10, 1-15.

Ownsworth, TL, McFarland, K., & Young RM (2002). The investigation of factors underlying deficits in self-awareness and self-regulation. *Brain Injury*, 16, 291-309.

Memory

After a brain injury
Written by: McKay Moore Sohlberg, Ph.D.

✓ understand different types of memory
✓ correct common myths about memory
✓ lessen the effects of memory problems

Memory Basics

Difficulties with memory after a brain injury can be very frustrating and confusing for the individual and for the family. They also pose challenges for caregivers, therapists and clinicians who are providing care and treatment.

Understanding the following three concepts will take you a long way toward understanding changes in memory after brain injury.

Concept 1: There are different types of memory and they rely on different systems within the brain.

The brain does not process all information in the same way. Different types of brain injuries or diseases can affect memory in different ways. For example, persons with memory difficulties caused by a lack of oxygen to the brain because of a near drowning or heart attack are likely to quickly forget what they are told or have done. The brain has trouble storing new information.

On the other hand, a person with damage to their frontal lobes of the brain from a car crash may be able to learn new information but be unable to retrieve it without prompting. This person may have difficulty organizing new information and retrieving previously stored information.

Here are some of the different types of memory that can be affected when the brain has been damaged by an illness or injury.

Episodic memory... This involves memory for events that are tied to a time and place. Examples of difficulty are not remembering what one did the previous day or not recalling a visit from a friend.

Semantic memory... This involves facts that a person learns over time. Learning phone numbers used on a daily basis or learning the state capitals or planets in the solar system are examples of semantic memory.

This type of memory is often less affected in people with brain injuries than episodic memory.

Procedural memory... This is memory for well established sequences of activity that often involve motor movement. The person does not have to consciously recall information as the activity is done automatically. Examples are operating a washing machine, riding a bicycle, or opening a computer program. This type of memory is often quite strong in people with brain injury and helps them in rehabilitation.

Sometimes people can learn new procedures with lots of practice and repetition, even though they may not be aware of it. For example, they may be shown how to use a cell phone and will learn to automatically press the right button when it rings. But if you ask if they know what button to push, they may say no.

Retrograde memory... This is memory for events in a person's life that occurred before the brain injury, such as a graduation, wedding or trip. Most people can remember things that occurred before their brain injury better than they can remember things that happened after their brain injury. Retrograde amnesia is the term used to describe damage to this autobiographical or very personal memory. It is relatively rare.

Concept 2: Memory is not an island.

Memory is closely tied to other processes in the brain that affect how we think and learn. For example, a person who has difficulty with attention and concentration is also likely to have difficulty with memory. Similarly, a person who has problems understanding language after a brain injury is likely to have difficulty remembering the content of conversations. Memory is a very complex process that involves many different areas and systems within the brain.

Memory is also linked to our emotions and physical condition. We all have selective memory and tend to remember certain types of information better than others. Motivation and interest improve everybody's memory. For example, a person may remember that you promised to make a favorite dessert but not remember to take out the trash! Fatigue and pain also affect systems that process information in the brain. We don't remember as efficiently when we are tired or not feeling well. Memory function in people with brain injuries is even more affected by emotional and physical states than in people without brain injuries.

Concept 3: *Many people with severe memory impairments learn or relearn information best when it is presented errorlessly rather than by trial and error learning.*

Research shows that people with severe memory impairments do not learn as well in a trial and error format. This is where people try and guess information and then are corrected as they make mistakes. Errors confuse the learning process.

It is more effective to tell the person the information to be remembered before asking the person to repeat it back to you. Then gradually increase the time between when you tell the person and ask the question. This seems odd, as in the beginning you are giving the person the answer to a question before you actually ask the question. However, this rehearsal pattern can allow people with even severe memory impairments to learn new facts.

Myths and Facts about Memory

People have many different ideas about how memory works and what may affect it. Here are some of the most common misunderstandings.

Myth 1: *My memory will not get better if I use my memory book because I won't exercise my brain.*

Using information from the past and anticipating events in the future exercises the brain better than trying to think of information that may or may not have been stored in memory. Organizing key information by using memory books, notes, or other strategies helps the brain form links and connections. This actually provides more memory rehabilitation than trying to test oneself.

Myth 2: *My husband only remembers what he wants to.*

Memory is very uneven. Different types of information are processed differently in the brain. Only some areas of the different memory systems in a person's brain may be impaired after a brain injury. Other areas may be undamaged. Everyone's memory is affected by many different physical and emotional factors.

Myth 3: *It is best to have a person try and encourage the person to think about a target memory fact, rather than help supply the information.*

Remember...errorless learning works best.

Myth 4: *A person who won't use or abandons a strategy or system is not cooperating and not trying to get better.*

There are lots of reasons a system may go awry. For example:

- The strategy may not be a good match for the person.
- The person may not have had enough practice.
- The person may have successfully used the strategy before, but needs repeated training, support and practice to begin using it again. (Have you ever fallen off your exercise plan?)
- The person may feel angry or depressed and is exerting control by refusing to do what is asked. Giving the person more information about the development and selection of a memory strategy or system may help.
- Or, a dozen other reasons...

Memory problems can have a deep impact on how a person functions and gets through the day. Understanding the nature of the problem, identifying priorities, and making an action plan that is doable can go a long way in reducing the frustration and increasing the abilities of a person with a brain injury.

Managing Memory Problems

This section has tips for survivors, caregivers, therapists and families with strategies for managing memory problems at home and in the community.

Tips on teaching strategies and organizing the environment...

These suggestions help reduce demands on a person's memory system. It is important to consider an individual's specific circumstances, the environment where the person lives, and personal preferences. Is the environment noisy or calm, organized or chaotic? Do the recommended strategies fit the way the person lives and interacts with others? What does the person think might help the most to carry out daily goals? Fitting memory strategies into a person's daily routines reduces the risk of forgetting and helps a person do more. Here are some examples of ideas. Their success will depend on finding a good match for the type of memory issue and the person's abilities.

✓ Create a communication center at home with a calendar and message space where everybody can check on what is going on and when.

✓ Organize office or kitchen space to store items and equipment. Create a place for everything. Label drawers or cupboards. Store items in assigned places.

✓ Check to make sure that everything is where it is supposed to be on a regular basis.

✓ Identify a memory system. This might be a planner with a daily to do list, a personal digital assistant (PDA), or a pager system that cues specific tasks. Make sure that the system chosen works for the person who will be using it. Some people do better with PDA's than paper. Other people find PDA's too complicated. Some people like a digital memory wrist watch. Fit the system to the person.

✓ Write down and post the steps or create checklists for specific tasks or activities such as laundry, grooming, or bill paying. Do this in locations where these activities occur. Post prompts of what a person needs to do around the house or work site so the person knows where to go to do the task.

✓ Use a backpack or tote bag to carry items needed for the day's activities. Put a checklist by the bag and keep it by the door. Remember, establishing a routine is key.

✓ Make a video or album with a personal story and include the person in its development. Encourage the person to refer to it regularly to help orientation.

✓ Reduce distractions whenever concentration or memory is required. Turn off the television and radio. Clean off the work space. Let people do one thing at a time.

Tips on using errorless learning approaches…

These can be used to teach information or strategies.

✓ Do not quiz a person on the information to be learned. Instead, begin by telling the key information to the person. Have the person repeat it. Then fade your prompt. For example, instead of saying, What is our address? try the following sequence:

Caregiver: Our address is 135 Marthas Court. Now you say it.

Individual: 135 Marthas Court.

✓ Repeat the sequence with more time between the caregiver's statement and the individual's response. Eventually the person will be able to give the information without first being given the answer. The idea is to try and prevent a person from guessing and giving a wrong answer that will later be remembered better than the corrected answer. Even people with severe memory impairments can learn new facts and procedures when information is presented errorlessly and with lots of repetition.

Tips on making information meaningful…

Make it special to the person by using these strategies.

✓ Link it to previous information that has been learned, or something that is important or of value to the person.

✓ Elaborate on information by using color coded checklists, pictures, putting information into a song or rhyme, and so on.

✓ Have the person say it again in their own words. This can make information more meaningful to anybody.

Tips on examining your expectations and setting priorities…

✓ Don't try to do everything at once.

✓ Take time to identify the most important memory issue you want to address and involve the person in this decision.

✓ Make a goal and remember that…
- It takes time to establish a routine.
- Everyone has ups and downs when learning how to use strategies.
- A person may benefit from occasional booster shots of support and reminders.

✓ Take time for yourself and ask for help.

Caregivers need respite or time off to provide ongoing support to others. If you are living with someone who has a severe memory impairment, you have a large responsibility. Make sure you take care of yourself.

Conclusion

Memory impairments are disruptive. However, understanding the complexity of memory and taking the time to try and implement strategies or systems can go a long way in lessening their effects. Those living with memory problems and those helping care for them are often in the best position to identify and evaluate the most effective strategies. It helps to start with practical ideas first. If they do not help, assistance from a teacher, speech and language pathologist or a psychologist who has experience working with people with brain injuries can also help.

Reference

Sohlberg, M. & Mateer, C. (2001). *Cognitive Rehabilitation: An integrative neuropsychological approach.* New York, NY: The Guilford Press.

Adults Living with Brain Injury

Written by: Carolyn Rocchio, Parent; Pam Fleming, CCC-SLP; & Erika Mountz, O.T.R./L.

✓ identify safety concerns
✓ encourage independence

Encouraging Independence

The first question after a person has a brain injury that many families ask is, When can he come home? This is often followed by... How will we manage? Can she be alone? How much supervision and help will he need?

It can be difficult to find the balance between protecting a person from further injury and encouraging independence. There are many factors to consider whether the person is just preparing to be discharged from the hospital or rehabilitation program or already living at home. This article provides checklists and strategies to guide families and caregivers. It can be used to identify areas where further treatment is needed, justify requests for services or funding, and improve the safety and independence of the person with a brain injury.

We all depend on others in some way, whether it is for physical help, emotional support, finances or learning. No matter how independent or dependent an individual is, we are all interdependent on others in some way.

Checklist for effects of brain injury on independence

Physical Changes

Does the person have...	always	mostly	sometimes	never
headaches	____	____	____	____
fatigue	____	____	____	____
seizures	____	____	____	____
sleep disorder	____	____	____	____
paralysis	____	____	____	____
one sided weakness	____	____	____	____
awkwardness or clumsiness	____	____	____	____
change/loss of taste and smell	____	____	____	____

Vision and Hearing

Is the person...	always	usually	sometimes	never
sensitive to noise	____	____	____	____
bothered by bright lights	____	____	____	____
affected by dizziness	____	____	____	____
able to hear on right side	____	____	____	____
able to hear on left side	____	____	____	____
have ringing in the ears	____	____	____	____
able to judge distance	____	____	____	____
able to judge height	____	____	____	____
able to see objects on left side	____	____	____	____
able to see objects on right side	____	____	____	____

Thinking and Learning

Can the person...	always	mostly	sometimes	never
pay attention and concentrate	____	____	____	____
get started in activities	____	____	____	____
break tasks into smaller steps	____	____	____	____
stick with a task until finished	____	____	____	____
concentrate with background noise	____	____	____	____
plan ahead	____	____	____	____
problem solve	____	____	____	____
learn new information	____	____	____	____
recall old information	____	____	____	____
make reasonable decisions	____	____	____	____
adjust to change	____	____	____	____
be flexible as things change	____	____	____	____

Behaviors, Awareness and Emotions

Can the person control....	always	mostly	sometimes	never
sexual comments	____	____	____	____
sexual gestures and actions	____	____	____	____
anger and avoid outbursts	____	____	____	____
physical aggression	____	____	____	____

Is the person...	always	mostly	sometimes	never
aware of strengths (intact abilities)	____	____	____	____
compensating for difficulties	____	____	____	____
lonely	____	____	____	____
depressed	____	____	____	____
hopeful about future	____	____	____	____

Living with brain injury

Self-Care

Can the person safely...	lots of help	some help	on own
take a bath or shower	____	____	____
brush teeth	____	____	____
use the toilet	____	____	____
organize belongings and room	____	____	____
find clothing and dress self	____	____	____
climb stairs	____	____	____
move over varied surfaces (carpeting, linoleum)	____	____	____
monitor personal hygiene	____	____	____
take medication	____	____	____

Orientation

Can the person...	lots of help	some help	on own
provide vital data, i.e. age, birthdate	____	____	____
give address and telephone number where living	____	____	____
give names and telephone numbers for emergencies	____	____	____
easily see and read clocks	____	____	____
name day of week and date	____	____	____

Communication

Can the person...	always	mostly	sometimes	never
speak clearly and be understood	____	____	____	____
use the telephone	____	____	____	____
write or print clearly	____	____	____	____
use a computer	____	____	____	____
understand written information	____	____	____	____

Home Safety

Does the person...	always	mostly	sometimes	never
remember to lock doors	____	____	____	____
remember to lock windows	____	____	____	____
know what to do in case of fire	____	____	____	____
know what to do in a power failure	____	____	____	____
limit personal info on telephone or Internet	____	____	____	____
stay home alone	____	____	____	____

Household

Can the person...	lots of help	some help	on own
separate, wash, dry and put away clothing	____	____	____
vacuum or sweep	____	____	____
determine if food is spoiled	____	____	____
plan and prepare a good meal	____	____	____
follow steps of a recipe	____	____	____
use stove safely	____	____	____
clean up after cooking	____	____	____
prepare menus	____	____	____
shop for food	____	____	____

Organization

Does the person...	lots of help	some help	on own
plan tasks and chores daily	____	____	____
plan appointments daily	____	____	____
set an alarm clock	____	____	____
wake and get up in morning	____	____	____

Social Skills

Can the person...	always	mostly	sometimes	never
fit in with peers	____	____	____	____
know what is expected in social situations	____	____	____	____
accept correction and/or supervision	____	____	____	____
use resources when needed	____	____	____	____
use leisure time productively	____	____	____	____
make appointments	____	____	____	____

Financial

Can the person...	lots of help	some help	on own
count money and make change	____	____	____
budget weekly and monthly	____	____	____
use a credit card	____	____	____
write checks	____	____	____
balance statements	____	____	____

Transportation

Is the person...	Yes	No
approved by a certified driving evaluation	___	___
safe to driving during the day	___	___
safe to drive at night	___	___

Is the person able to...	lots of help	some help	on own
use a public bus or subway	___	___	___
travel by plane	___	___	___
get and pay for a taxi	___	___	___
go for local walks	___	___	___

Risk factors

Is the person a user of...	often	sometimes	never
alcohol	___	___	___
"street" drugs	___	___	___

Legal issues

Does the person...	Yes	No
have a guardian or conservator	___	___
receive government benefits	___	___
responsibly manage benefits or insurance funds	___	___
have plans for the future to prevent loss of benefits	___	___
have all important papers and applications up to date and stored in one place	___	___

Strategies for protection, changing behavior and personal safety

Tips for protecting others from out of control behavior...
✓ Model calm when the person is out of control.
✓ Remove oneself from the presence of the out of control person.
✓ Do not try to defuse the situation until calm is reached.

Tips for changing behavior...
✓ Video tape unwanted behavior for later discussion.
✓ Draw up behavioral contracts with rewards for good behavior.
✓ Avoid focusing on negative behaviors and praise positive behaviors.
✓ Rehearse appropriate behavior before attending public functions.

Tips for personal safety...
✓ Have identification on the person all the time.
✓ Have an action plan if the smoke detector or burglar alarm goes off.
✓ Carry medical information, ie. medic alert emblem, bracelet or wallet card.
✓ Lay out a safe route for walking or jogging when alone.
✓ Have the person medically cleared before doing any balance activities such as biking, skating, roller blading.
✓ Determine if the person has sufficient insight about difficulties to safely try new activities.

✓ Provide one on one monitoring until a skill is safely mastered.

Conclusion

You can use these checklists at any stage of a person's recovery to chart progress and to identify improvements leading to greater independence.

Prior to discharge - If the person whom you expect to provide care for has not been discharged yet, share this checklist with therapists who are familiar with the individual. This will give you a baseline or starting point to track progress after the person comes home or enters another program.

After discharge - If you are caring for or supervising an individual who no longer has therapies regularly, include the individual and family members in the discussion. It is important that everyone providing care agree on the individual's current level of skill and decision making abilities. This information can be used to identify short and long term goals to promote a greater independence.

Copyright © 2008 by Lash & Associates Publishing/Training Inc.
This material is copyrighted by Lash & Associates and can not be reproduced in any form without permission.
Lash & Associates Publishing/Training Inc.
Tel. & Fax (919) 562-0015 or visit our web site *www.lapublishing.com*
This article is not intended as a substitute for the medical advice of your physician. Consult your doctor regularly about matters concerning your health, particularly regarding symptoms that require diagnosis or immediate medical attention.

Social Skills

After brain injury
Written by: Harvey E. Jacobs, Ph.D.

✓ explains importance of social skills
✓ identifies receiving and sending skills
✓ addresses challenges for social skills

What are Social Skills?

Alex is hilarious; at least he thinks so, though no one else seems to get his jokes, no matter how many times he tells them over and over and over again.

Pauline doesn't understand why her boss is angry with her for whooping it up at work this morning. After all, everybody was pretty crazy at the company picnic this weekend, so what is the problem with bringing some fun back to the job?

Betty can't understand why she can't get a date. It's not for lack of trying, and she is attractive. She's even gotten to the point of asking people out when she first meets them.

Each of these individuals has challenges with social skills. What does this mean? Social skills are the behaviors that people see and show when interacting with others. This includes what people say or do, their posture, and their physical location. It also includes their manner of dress, their tone and volume of voice. It is almost anything that is conveyed between people. Social skills cover just about everything that we do or say. Consider your own social skills!

Some social situations are fairly stable and the rules for social skills rarely change. For example, you probably have a basic way that you interact with your boss at work. However, the rules and expectations for social skills can vary greatly in dynamic situations. What may be acceptable behavior in one social situation may not work in another, or can even change within a situation. For example, consider how rapidly events change at a busy party. You may be speaking to one person one minute and someone else the next. Topics of conversation can quickly change depending on who is around. It's also important to be able to "read the party" and know whether to stay or leave.

Successful Social Skills

Being successful in social situations involves multi-tasking. This is the ability to use many different skills at the same time. Most of these skills can be broken down into *receiving skills* and *sending skills*.

Receiving skills are the ability to read and understand the current social situation. This includes recognizing...

- *Which people are involved in the situation* –
  Can the person identify who is involved, who is an observer, or who is not involved in the situation?

- *The topic or theme of the social situation* –
  Does the person know the purpose of the situation; for example, is it business, polite chat, problem solving, humor, sarcastic bantering, or an intimate discussion?

- *Information being discussed* –
  Does the person understand the flow of the situation?

- *The person's role* –
  Is the person a key participant, a polite listener, or not even part of the situation?

- *Reactions to the person* –
  Do people pay attention, encourage, ignore, or "suffer" the person politely?

Dynamic receiving skills involve the ability to continually read the flow of the social situation. Being able to "go with the flow" is critical because social situations are constantly changing. This requires fluid and adaptive thinking. To be socially successful, a person has to be able to:

- Follow the course of a conversation
- Change focus as topics change
- Be aware of other events going on, such as people joining or leaving the setting.

Sending skills focus on how a person presents himself (sends himself) to others.

Non-verbal sending skills include:

- *Basic abilities such as grooming and personal hygiene*
  It's important to prepare for the occasion, whether it is overalls on the farm or a suit for a job interview.

- *Personal distance between people*
  This varies by culture and situation. The average personal distance in the US is about three feet. This can change with the situation, such as during an intimate conversation, when on an airplane, or standing in an elevator.

- *Body language*
  This includes posture, gestures, eye contact, and movements. These often send more information to the recipient (listener) than what is actually said, especially to strangers. Consider how little you actually hear from someone if you feel threatened.

Verbal sending skills involve how and what a person says. Not only is what a person says important, but so is the person's tone, volume, pitch, timing and clarity. It is also important to know what not to say!

Challenges for Social Skills after Brain Injury

Many people have challenges with social skills after a brain injury for a variety of reasons. Some of the greatest challenges may include:

Context

Having fewer social opportunities is usually more of a barrier to successful social interaction than the brain injury itself. Not returning to military duty or work often means that a person loses contact with people who were once an important part of a social support network. Being unable to keep up with friends and comrades may lead to loneliness and isolation. Changes in roles and relationships at home can produce similar problems. These changes can be difficult for anyone, but having a brain injury can make this more stressful. The challenge is how to create positive and meaningful social opportunities for everyone involved.

Problems of production and reception

Problems with speech can include changes in...

- producing words and sentences
- speaking clearly

- rising or falling pitch of the voice
- understanding what is said or read
- hearing

Any of these can make it more challenging for a person to interact with other people. Adaptive devices such as spelling or word boards, synthesized speaking machines, etc., may help but they may slow the natural flow of conversation in social situations.

Self-concept and emotions

Interacting with others can be challenging if you feel bad about yourself or believe that others see you negatively. After a brain injury, many people withdraw from social situations because they feel unable to keep up or believe that others do not value them. Some people feel depressed or overwhelmed, while others report agitation or frustration. Sometimes the person with a brain injury expresses little emotion or has less interest in interacting with anybody. Changes in frustration levels or temperament may result in avoidance by others.

When a person feels unable to fit in or has a bad social experience, it can be embarrassing and the person may react with feelings of shame. It is important for others to help the person understand what has happened, learn what skills are needed and to encourage the person to continue working on social skills.

Self-centeredness

Some people become very self-centered (egocentric) after a brain injury. They may have little interest in others or are unable to see another person's viewpoints. When problems occur, they may not be aware of the difficulty or assume that it is someone else's fault. Others may avoid people with this self-centered behavior because of the frustrations when trying to communicate with them.

Awareness and social perception

Lack of awareness to social situations or the social cues of others is often reported in persons with brain injuries. Sometimes this is due to difficulty concentrating during a long period of social contact. Other times, there are problems with poor attention to detail or the inability to read the fine details of the social situation. These problems can cause misunderstandings. Sometimes people simply lose the ability to monitor their behavior or the behavior of others after a brain injury.

Other challenges

People may have many other challenges when trying to navigate social situations. Physical changes in mobility, coordination, walking, and endurance may make it difficult for persons to be in social situations after a brain injury. Fatigue may make it harder for a person to think clearly and interact with others. Changes in vision, hearing, or damage to other senses may affect how people understand and interpret basic information. Other cognitive and memory challenges can make it harder for a person to remember or follow the current conversation, or to follow up on previous conversations. Increased or decreased arousal can cause a person to come on too strong or too timidly. None of these issues occurs in isolation. Rather, how each person acts socially is usually a combination of these factors.

What to Do

It is hard for most people to receive negative feedback, so it is important to provide support carefully and with compassion. Sometimes people are able to develop new skills to overcome these challenges after brain injury. Other times, they may need help (supports) to manage the situation, including someone serving as an "interpreter" to help them understand the situation.

Tips for helping in social situations...
✓ Remember that social skills are no different than any other skills.
✓ Take the shame out of a problem situation.
✓ Focus on the practical and the factual, rather than the emotional.
✓ Emphasize the positive over the negative – what a person can do over what can't be done.

Some social situations may be too overwhelming for the person or the person may be too overwhelming for the social situation. The worst decision is to simply exclude someone from a situation, especially if it is important to the person. Of course, there may be times when this is necessary, but this should be the exception and not the rule!

Tips for finding ways for the person to be successful in social situations...
✓ Build skills in less demanding situations first and then transition to desired settings.
✓ Role-play or practice skills ahead of time.
✓ Be an interpreter, not the voice, to help the person use his/her words and actions.
✓ Determine if the problems are related to sending or receiving skills and then practice these skills one by one before combining them for more complex situations.

Sending skills are often easier to teach than receiving skills.

Tips for teaching sending skills...
✓ Role play to practice social distance, tone of voice, dress, and length of discussion.
✓ Videotape these sessions for review.
✓ Start with the basics, then work up to the more difficult.
✓ Give more support to people in more complex social situations.

Receiving skills usually involve judgment and perception. If a person is "pretty good" at receiving skills, but just needs a little more polish, you can ask the person to describe an actual situation and give corrections. In other cases, it may be necessary to use different teaching and compensatory techniques.

Tips for teaching receiving skills...
✓ Videotape the person in simulated situations to provide feedback on performance.
✓ Focus on the person's interpretation of what was going on during the replay.
✓ Ask the person to watch others in social situations and analyze their performance. (Television and movies are a great way to do this.)
✓ Have a person who does well verbally in social situations but has difficulty with non-verbal aspects watch television with the sound off and explain what is going on with people's emotions, body language, personal distance, dress, etc. (Soap operas are great for this.)

Many individuals report feeling socially isolated because of the effects of the brain injury and the changes in their lives. This can lead to boredom, frustration, loneliness, lowered self-esteem and depression. Support groups for persons with brain injury are a place for giving and receiving emotional support, sharing information, and reducing isolation. Support groups are run by state affiliates of the Brain Injury Association of America and by many hospital and rehabilitation programs.

Find a Mentor

People who have greater difficulty understanding social situations may benefit from "mentors" who can cue them. Mentors are usually people who are close to the individual and can also be in the social setting. This may include friends or family members who the individual is willing to receive feedback from. Using pre-arranged signals, the mentor can help the individual know when to start or stop talking, when it is time to leave, re-establish personal space, and so on.

Finally, there may be some times when the person is not be able to navigate social situations successfully. This can be difficult, especially if the person wants to be involved. Frank and supportive discussion may be needed to address the issue. If this does not work, then help from more experienced people or professionals may build success.

Conclusion

Our social skills are always on display every day as the situation and setting change. While a number of challenges may affect successful social skills following a brain injury, many of these issues can be overcome with training and compassionate support.

References

Ownsworth, T.L., McFarland, R., Young, D. (2000). Self-awareness and psychosocial functioning following acquired brain injury: An evaluation of a group support programme. Neur*opsychological Rehabilitation*10(5): 465-484.

Snow, P, Douglas, J, Ponsford, J. (2000). Conversational assessment following traumatic brain injury: A comparison across two control groups. *Brain Injury* 11(6):465-484.

Aging
With a Brain Injury
Written by: Mary Hibbard, Ph.D.

✓ correct common misunderstandings
✓ provide updated information
✓ make changes for healthy living

Growing Older

More individuals who have survived a brain injury are getting older. Many are concerned about the long-term effects of their brain injury and fear a further decline in thinking abilities or worry about developing Alzheimer's disease. Others worry about having another brain injury. Studies about the long-term effects of brain injury are just beginning, so there are many unanswered questions.

Concerns

"My memory was poor after my brain injury. It seems to be getting worse now as I get older. Will my memory continue to decline as I age?"

"Making decisions was much harder after my brain injury. But now that I am getting older, my ability to make decisions is even worse."

Facts

Almost everybody has natural declines in thinking and problem solving with aging. Typical complaints are worsening memory, slowed responses, difficulty concentrating, and trouble thinking flexibly – especially in new situations.

These "normal" changes with aging add to the challenges of a person with a brain injury. Some individuals with brain injury report they have more cognitive (thinking and learning) difficulties as they get older. Others are less aware of changes, yet families report losses in the person's overall functioning. Some individuals have called these changes "premature aging after brain injury".

Any major life change can affect cognitive abilities as the person ages with a brain injury. Sudden changes in familiar routines such as loss of work or a marital separation or divorce can be especially difficult. Other major life changes can include deaths of close family or friends.

With aging, the person may use more drugs or alcohol, have side effects of medication prescribed for other age related illnesses, be under more stress, feel socially isolated and have declines in general mood.

Cognitive tips for persons aging with brain injury...

✓ Use schedules, notebooks, memory organizers and calendars regularly. They help a person stay organized after a brain injury and are even more essential as a person ages (even for people without a brain injury).

✓ Keep day-to-day activities as structured and predictable as possible to help overall thinking abilities.

✓ Reduce stimulation and distractions. This will help concentration and thinking abilities.

✓ Keep your mind active with mental exercises and social stimulation. The saying, "If you don't use it, you lose it" applies to the brain as well as muscles in the body as a person ages.

✓ Have healthy eating habits. The brain needs nourishment to function properly.

✓ Develop a routine aerobic exercise program. Exercise improves thinking abilities and mood as well as fitness and well-being.

✓ Avoid using illegal drugs or alcohol. They worsen thinking, judgment, memory and reasoning skills.

✓ Schedule routine checkups to monitor physical health and wellness. A medical illness may reduce thinking abilities.

✓ Monitor mood and seek professional help if becoming depressed or anxious. Depression and anxiety can reduce thinking and concentration abilities.

Concern

"Ever since I had my brain injury, I worry that I will end up with Alzheimer's disease when I get older."

Facts

Current research has no definitive answers. Some studies suggest that a brain injury places a person at greater risk of developing Alzheimer's disease with aging. Other research fails to support this. There are two risk factors for the development of Alzheimer's disease that are unrelated to brain injury. The first is a family history of Alzheimer's disease. The second is the presence of a specific genetic marker, called apolipoprotein E (APOE 4).

Some research indicates that individuals with brain injury, who have one or both of these risk factors, may be at increased risk of developing Alzheimer's disease at a younger age than peers with the same risks but no prior brain injury. This finding is controversial. More research is needed to better understand the specific risks for Alzheimer's disease following brain injury.

Alzheimer's disease is often difficult to diagnose in older adults. Other factors often mimic the disease. Reduced thinking abilities from a prior brain injury may be further affected by declines in thinking abilities with aging. This can result in the person functioning *as if* Alzheimer's disease were developing - but the person actually does not have the disease.

Other possible reasons for declines in thinking and overall functioning include a new medical condition, poor nutrition, a new neurological illness (such as a stroke or another brain injury), onset of a severe depression, interactions between medications, or a poor reaction to a new medication. Important factors for a correct diagnosis are careful review of a person's physical and emotional state, prior family history, and a look at how the person's functioning has changed over time.

Medical tips for persons aging with brain injury...

✓ Seek medical attention for any marked change in thinking, functioning or physical health. Avoiding professional attention only results in unnecessary health risks since many medical situations are reversible.

✓ Get help from professionals knowledgeable about normal aging and the impact of brain injury on aging. They include neurologists (doctors specializing in neurological disorders), physiatrists (doctors specializing in physical rehabilitation), neuropsychologists (psychologists specializing in treatment of individuals with brain injury) and/or gerontologists (doctors specializing in aging).

✓ Tell any professional providing treatment about a prior brain injury, general functioning since the brain injury, and ANY RECENT changes. Bring copies of medical records related to the earlier brain injury including any reports of prior thinking abilities.

✓ Seek additional rehabilitation services if a diagnosis of Alzheimer's disease is made. Cognitive remediation and emotional support, as well as medications, may help.

✓ Keep up with current research about new medications and health supplements that may help minimize further loss of memory or functioning. Consult with a physician *before* taking them.

Concern

"Does having one brain injury mean that I am more likely to have another brain injury as I age?"

Facts

A person with one brain injury is three times more likely to have a second brain injury. Individuals with two brain injuries are ten times more likely to have a third injury. Repeated brain injuries result in cumulative damage to the brain. This means that the effects build up over time with each repeated injury. This may result in poorer physical, thinking and emotional functioning.

Changes in thinking abilities - such as trouble concentrating, distractibility, impulsiveness and poor judgment - can all result in another injury. Physical changes such as poor balance, dizziness, slowed motor speed, sensory changes, seizures, sleep disturbances and pain can also increase the risks.

Falls pose a serious health risk and are the most common reasons for brain injury in older adults. The risk of falling is even greater for older individuals with a prior brain injury due to reductions in thinking and physical agility as a person ages.

Safety tips for persons aging with brain injury...

✓ Protect the head to avoid repeated brain injuries.

✓ Avoid action sports that can increase the odds of another brain injury.

- ✓ Use protective headgear when biking, skating, and playing baseball or other sports.

- ✓ Wear a seat belt in a car or other moving vehicle - *always*.

- ✓ Avoid events requiring rapid physical response or agility if these skills were affected by the first brain injury. They tend to become more problematic with aging.

- ✓ Stop and review options in a new situation and choose the best response BEFORE reacting. Individuals with brain injury often have difficulty stopping impulsive actions. Accidents are more likely to occur when people do things impulsively.

- ✓ Minimize involvement in stimulating activities when tired. Fatigue will only reduce thinking abilities and response time, thus increasing the risk of accidents.

- ✓ Ensure that home, work and community places are safe, well lit and fall-proof.

- ✓ Continue taking prescribed medications according to the doctor's instructions, especially if there is a seizure disorder. There is increased risk of a repeated brain injury if a seizure occurs and a person loses balance, falls or loses consciousness.

Concern

"Will my life span be shortened because of my brain injury?"

Facts

Research on this topic is limited. In general, older individuals and those with more severe injuries are less likely to survive initially. People who have a brain injury later in life are also likely to experience more handicaps and a poorer quality of life than younger adults, regardless of the severity of their initial injuries. Those who survive at least one year after more severe brain injuries have only slightly shorter life expectancies than people without brain injury. Individuals with mild brain injury have only slightly shorter life expectancies than peers without brain injury.

Lifestyle tips for persons aging with brain injury...

- ✓ Assume you will live to old age and plan accordingly!

- ✓ Maintain a healthy lifestyle as you age with your brain injury. This will help minimize age related medical conditions which may shorten your life span.

- ✓ Avoid repeated injury to your brain.

Concern

"I already rely on others to help me with everyday tasks. What will happen when I am older...will I need to plan for additional help?"

"Since my brain injury in my early twenties, I have lived with my parents. They help me do many things in the community. I am worried about my parents dying and what will become of me after they are gone."

Facts

Most individuals with disabilities (including those with brain injury) are living longer and live in the community. An individual with physical disabilities may need help with personal skills such as bathing and dressing by family members or paid assistants. But by far the greatest challenges for most persons with brain injuries are the less visible (but life long) disabilities in thinking, memory, personality and emotional control. While help may be willingly provided by family, friends or hired aides early in recovery, this may change over time. The social isolation of many further limits options for help. Insurance benefits for home based services are often time limited and discontinued long before the need has ended. These trends suggest the importance of long term planning to ensure the best possible quality of life as persons age with brain injury.

Planning tips for persons aging with brain injury...

- ✓ Know your health care benefits and advocate for services you need.

- ✓ Explore eligibility for government funded programs for persons with disability and/or brain injury in your state, such as the brain injury waiver program and Section 8 housing. Such programs typically have long waiting lists, so it is best to place your name on it as soon as possible.

- ✓ Discuss long term planning with your family and support circle. Have a frank discussion of your current challenges and help needed (now and in the future). Talk about possible living arrangements and finances for the future.

- ✓ Identify a person to be your health care proxy. This person should be willing to serve as your future advocate and help you make decisions as you age. Keep that person involved in your long term plans.

- ✓ Consider talking with a lawyer for planning financial support in the future. Choose one familiar with disability and elder care law.

Conclusion

The normal aging process can be challenging for individuals with brain injury. It is important to maintain wellness, maximize healthy living, prevent repeated brain injures and minimize risks of other age related diseases.

References

Aravich, PF, McDonnell AM (2005). Successful Aging of Individuals with Brain Injury. *Brain Injury/Professional* 2(2), 10-14.

Flanagan S, Hibbard MR, Gordon WA (2005). The impact of age on traumatic brain injury. *Physical Medicine and Rehabilitation Clinics of North America* 16, 163-177.

Substance Abuse
Prevention and Treatment After Brain Injury
Written by: John D. Corrigan, Ph.D. & Roberta DePompei, Ph.D.

✓ identifies signs of substance abuse
✓ explains reasons for substance abuse
✓ gives information on prevention, education and interventions

What is Substance Abuse?

Substance abuse and substance dependence are two *substance use disorders*. They are different than being intoxicated. With disorders, there are physical, cognitive or social consequences for the person using alcohol or other drugs. It is important to distinguish between the use of alcohol and other drugs and their *misuse*.

Any use of alcohol and other drugs by a person with a brain injury can slow recovery, worsen symptoms, interact with prescribed medications, or even increase the possibility of seizures.

Substance use and brain injury

There are many reasons why substance use and traumatic brain injury often go together.

- *Alcohol or illicit drugs were used before the injury.* Habits of drug use are hard to change and resuming previous use is common. It is even harder if peers, friends or relatives drink or use other drugs.

- *Drug and alcohol use can develop after a brain injury.* Adjusting to a disability is stressful. Frustration, anger, and sorrow are natural reactions to losses and changes caused by brain injury. Turning to substances may be an attempt by the person to "feel better".

- *Tolerance levels of substances are decreased.* The person becomes high faster and longer after a brain injury, regardless of prior patterns of substance use. A smaller quantity of chemicals can produce a magnified, uncharacteristic effect which may feel pleasurable to the person.

- *Ability to self-monitor appropriate social behavior is decreased.* The person's ability to use cognitive skills (thinking, planning, organizing, problem solving) to monitor the social consequences of behaviors is often affected by a brain injury. The person may erroneously conclude that the effects of drugs or alcohol are not a problem.

- *Social groups change.* When old friends are lost, the person with a brain injury may look for new peers to avoid feeling lonely. If the new group uses substances, they may be more willing to tolerate unusual and inappropriate social behaviors by the person with a brain injury.

- *Pain or potential seizure activity after an injury may require prescription drugs.* The increased availability of prescription drugs can become a problem if the person uses more than the prescribed dose to get high.

How Do You Know There's a Problem?

Professionals can increase the amount and accuracy of information gathered by...

- Being alert to risk factors and signs of substance abuse.

- Trying to be non-judgmental when discussing drugs or alcohol use.

- Establishing a trusting relationship.

- Keeping conversation at a level suitable for the age, cultural background and cognitive abilities of the person with a brain injury.

Ask and listen

Ask the person to tell you about an issue rather than rapidly firing questions. The following topics are not a list of questions to be posed one after another; they are guidelines for conversations about drug and alcohol use.

Tips for professionals...

✓ *Ask what drugs are being used and how much.*

Listen for whether the person is using more than one drug, if the goal is to get high, if amounts used are increasing, or if the type of drug is changing to keep getting high.

✓ *Ask about history of use.*

Listen for age when alcohol or other drugs were first tried, whether there was counseling or other treatment, and if the person was under the influence of drugs when injured.

✓ *Ask about effects of use.*

Listen for indications of family or peer difficulties arising from use, legal or financial consequences, problems on duty, at school or work, physical problems, or emotional consequences.

✓ *Ask about social context of use.*

Listen for whether and how much friends or family are using, the extent to which activities are planned around use, or whether the person feels unable to relax and socialize without using.

✓ *Ask about family's history of use and/or abuse.*

Listen for substance abuse problems in the immediate family or biological relatives and the extent to which family activities or get-togethers regularly involve substance use.

If listening reveals potential problems in more than one of the above areas, there is most likely a substance use problem and action is needed.

What to Do if You Suspect a Problem

Careful listening by family members helps when discussing substance misuse. Discuss any concerns with a professional who is working with you.

Tips for families...

✓ *Don't panic.*

You must keep calm to help the person who is struggling with these problems.

✓ *Tap resources to inform yourself.*

There is help and support available from your national or state brain injury association. They know of groups that deal with disabilities and substance abuse.

✓ *Get a referral.*

Talk with your physician or case manager to set up a referral to a local drug and alcohol program or clinic where you can obtain education, assistance, or treatment.

✓ *Use a "NO USE" message.*

Everyone involved with the individual must agree there will be no use of alcohol or drugs in any form. This includes family occasions where "just one glass of beer or wine" is served and social discussions where alcohol or persons who use it are considered heroes.

Intervention

A substance abuse professional can determine the level of care needed depending on the severity of a person's problem. Common treatment settings include detoxification programs, residential treatment, intensive outpatient care, and counseling. Treatment may involve one or more of the following: self-help groups, 12-step programs, family therapy, education, cognitive-behavioral psychotherapy, or psycho-pharmacology. The more severe the problem, the more time it takes to establish new and healthy behaviors.

Prevention

Anyone with a brain injury needs education about substance use. Sooner or later, each person faces decisions about whether to use drugs and alcohol after his or her traumatic brain injury. Because judgment and problem solving can be affected, individuals with brain injuries may be more susceptible to opportunities to use. Providing information and support can help them make good decisions. Educate early and often about the problems of alcohol and other drugs after brain injury.

A True/False quiz was developed by the Ohio Valley Center for Brain Injury Prevention and Rehabilitation.

T F   People who use alcohol or other drugs after they have a brain injury don't recover as much.

T F   Brain injuries cause problems in balance, walking or talking that get worse when a person uses alcohol or other drugs.

T F   People who have had a brain injury often say or do things without thinking first, a problem that is made worse by using alcohol and other drugs.

T F   Brain injuries cause problems with thinking, like concentration or memory, and using alcohol or other drugs makes these problems worse.

T F   After brain injury, alcohol and other drugs have a more powerful effect.

T F   People who have had a brain injury are more likely to have times that they feel low or depressed and drinking alcohol and getting high on other drugs makes this worse.

T F   After a brain injury, drinking alcohol or using other drugs can cause a seizure.

T F   People who drink alcohol or use other drugs after a brain injury are more likely to have another brain injury.

There are eight questions, but just one correct answer: TRUE. It's also true that the only amount of alcohol or other drugs that is safe to use after brain injury is NONE.

Conclusion

The potential for use of substances in persons with brain injuries is always present. Being alert to the reasons for substance abuse, warning signs, and possible behaviors that can develop will help families and professionals recognize a problem. Prevention, education, support, and referral can help minimize long-term effects. A list of resources follows.

Resources

Brain Injury Association
Family Helpline: 1-800-444-6443;
http://www.biausa.org

Al-Anon-AlTeen
http://www.al-anon.alateen.org

Just Say No International
http://www.justsayno.org/

National Clearinghouse for Alcohol and Drug Information
http://www.health.org

Ohio Valley Center for Brain Injury Prevention and Rehabilitation
http://www.ohiovalley.org

References

Corrigan, J.D., Bogner, J.A. & Lamb-Hart, G. L. Substance abuse and brain injury (1999). In M. Rosenthal, E.R. Griffith, J.D Miller and J. Kreutzer (Eds.) *Rehabilitation of the Adult and Child with Traumatic Brain Injury,* 3rd Edition. Philadelphia, PA: F.A. Davis Co.

DePompei, R., & Weis, J. (1996). Substance abuse and families of children with ABI. In G. Singer, A. Glang, and J. Williams (Eds.) *Children with acquired brain injury,* p. 167-187. Baltimore, MD: Paul H. Brookes Publishing Co.

Corrigan, J.D., Lamb-Hart G.L. (2004). *Substance Abuse Issues after Traumatic Brain Injury.* McLean, VA: Brain Injury Association of America.

Going to College or Technical School
After a brain injury
Written by: Jane E. B. Goodwin, M.A., CCC-SLP & Linda E. Larson, M.A., CCC-SLP

✓ explains federal laws
✓ describes academic accommodations
✓ gives strategies for learning

Going to College or Technical School?

Finding the right program can be an exciting and fun experience. However, it can become very complicated and frustrating if you are one of the many who has had a brain injury.

By collecting information, seeking appropriate accommodations and using compensatory strategies, students with brain injuries or other disabilities can succeed in college or technical school. It is important for veterans and vocational rehabilitation counselors to take the initiative to develop supports in the college or technical school setting.

Federal Laws can Help

Two pieces of federal legislation directly influence the Special Services Programs at universities and colleges. These programs are designed to help students with disabilities or special needs.

Section 504 of the Rehabilitation Act of 1973 states that "no otherwise qualified disabled individual can be denied access to, or participation in, any federally funded activity or program solely on the basis of disability...." This means that any college receiving federal funds can not exclude a qualified applicant or student only because of a disability.

Americans with Disabilities Act, Public Law 101-336 was signed in July 1990. This law extends the prohibition against discrimination on the basis of disability in Section 504 to all programs, activities and services provided or made available by state and local governments, regardless of whether those entities receive federal financial assistance. The law, often referred to as the ADA, requires accommodations to be reasonable and timely. It is often referred to as the civil rights law for persons with disabilities.

Under the ADA, the term "disability" means that an individual has a physical or mental impairment that substantially limits one or more major activities; has a record of the impairment; or is regarded as having an impairment.

What is a Reasonable Accommodation?

Title 1 of the ADA deals with Employment Provisions. It classifies a reasonable accommodation as "any modification or adjustment to a job, employment practice or a work environment that makes it possible for a qualified individual with a disability to participate in and enjoy an equal opportunity." The same applies to universities and colleges.

A potential student must meet academic criteria for admission. The presence of a disability does not change the academic requirements. In order for a person to seek assistance with any aspect of college admission, class accessibility or academic settings, the person must be willing to disclose the disability and provide clinical documentation of a disability.

Special Services in College

For the veteran who has a brain injury, or anyone with a disability, it is important to identify what resources, accommodations and supports will be available not only during the admissions process but once the student is enrolled.

Tips on questions to ask about applications and admissions...
✓ Who can help with the application process?
✓ Who has information about financial aid?
✓ What documentation of the disability is required? By whom - doctor, psychiatrist, psychologist, etc.?
✓ Is priority registration allowed?
✓ Are reduced course loads permitted?

Explore other services, find out if the college has...

- a tutoring center - if not, how are individual tutors arranged?
- academic counselors who specialize in working with students who have disabilities
- study skills or time management workshops held on campus
- a center or individuals who can assist with writing skills
- support group for students with disabilities
- map which shows handicapped features (bathrooms, elevators, parking, ramps, curb cuts)
- handicapped housing
- foreign language requirement waiver.

Academic Accommodations

Tips on exams...

- ✓ Can exam times be extended?
- ✓ Can a distraction free environment be arranged?
- ✓ Is it possible to have a reader for test questions?
- ✓ Is it possible to arrange a scribe to write exams to dictation (if the student has poor hand functioning)?
- ✓ Are oral tests vs. written tests available?
- ✓ Can print format be altered for impaired vision?

Tips on lectures...

- ✓ Is it possible to obtain a syllabus before class starts?
- ✓ Can note takers or note buddies be arranged?
- ✓ Can lectures be audiotaped?
- ✓ Can preferential seating be arranged?

Tips on classroom assignments...

- ✓ Is it possible to extend due dates?
- ✓ Can meetings with professors be arranged to assist with project planning?
- ✓ Can text readers be arranged?

Helping the Student Learn

Brain injuries can result in difficulties with cognitive (thinking) skills such as:

- attention and concentration
- memory
- information processing
- reasoning and problem solving
- executive functions (initiation, planning, insight, etc.)

These changes can make it difficult, but not impossible, to learn. Some of the following techniques may help.

Speech and Language

Tips on reading comprehension...

- ✓ highlight passages with a colored marker
- ✓ use a straight edge to stay on the line
- ✓ preview chapter summary prior to reading
- ✓ get books on tape
- ✓ take notes while reading
- ✓ read information aloud
- ✓ limit reading to 15 minute blocks

Tips on auditory comprehension...

- ✓ sit in front of class
- ✓ bring textbook to class
- ✓ develop outline from lecture
- ✓ tape lecture
- ✓ copy all information off the board
- ✓ ask for clarification of information

Tips on verbal language...

- ✓ speak loudly and clearly
- ✓ prepare questions ahead of time
- ✓ keep comments on topic
- ✓ use gestures or writing to help communicate

Tips on written language...

- ✓ get a note taker
- ✓ use a personal computer
- ✓ take oral vs. written tests
- ✓ develop an outline from the lecture
- ✓ get assistance with proofreading

Cognition or Thinking and Learning

Tips on information organizers...

- ✓ use an assignment notebook
- ✓ use a 3-ring binder or folder with pockets
- ✓ date notes
- ✓ develop a "to do" list

Tips on study time...

- ✓ avoid cramming
- ✓ schedule study time
- ✓ find quiet study space
- ✓ schedule study breaks
- ✓ avoid distractions
- ✓ break projects down into smaller steps

Tips on study techniques...

✓ color code similar information
✓ highlight notes
✓ use index cards as flashcards
✓ join study groups
✓ get a study partner
✓ ask for feedback on performance

Conclusion

It is important to work with your vocational rehabilitation counselor when considering all your options for making a successful transition in college or other technical school setting. Don't get in over your head. You might want to talk to your vocational rehabilitation counselor about starting with a part time program or just one course. Many local community colleges have well established programs to accommodate students with special needs. The bottom line is to keep your expectations reasonable. It's much better to start off slowly and gradually increase the academic load as you adjust to your new setting. Build a support system, use the services available, and maximize your opportunities to succeed.

Resources

Vet Success
www.vetsuccess.gov

References

Roberts Stoler, D. & Albers Hill, B. (1998). *Coping with Mild Traumatic Brain Injury.* Garden City Park, NY: Avery Publishing Group.

Americans with Disabilities Act
http://www.usdoj.gov/crt/ada/adahom1.htm

US Dept Health and Human Services, Office for Civil Rights

http://www.hhs.gov/ocr/504.html

Adults with Brain Injury

Myths and Stereotypes About Work and Life

Written by: Jeffrey S. Kreutzer, Ph.D., ABPP & Stephanie A. Kolakowsky-Hayner, M.A.

✓ shows how stereotypes develop
✓ examines beliefs about people with disabilities
✓ discusses negative stereotypes

Common Stereotypes

Stereotypes are widely held ideas or beliefs that are dangerous because they are often unfair, false, fail to recognize individual differences, show great disrespect, or translate into negative attitudes. They usually arise from misinformation or lack of information. Persons with disabilities have often been the subject of stereotypes and described as...

- sinister or evil
- having superpowers
- laughable
- non-sexual
- bitter and isolated
- a burden on others

Myths about Brain Injury

The general public is rarely given factual information about brain injury and its consequences. Most people form ideas about brain injury from television, magazines, and newspapers. The press tends to focus on positive stories, for example, describing people who've had miraculous recoveries or accomplished miraculous feats.

More than ten million people read tabloid newspapers regularly. Tabloids sell by printing sensational stories. Recent stories about the brain and brain injury include...

- Transplanting brains and heads from people to animals and vice versa
- Keeping human heads alive for months or years while awaiting transplant to animals or human bodies
- People awakening from a coma speaking new foreign languages or having other advanced skills
- Heads exploding from too much concentrating and thinking.

A far greater audience has been exposed to cartoons and slapstick comedy. The idea that people are "hard-headed" has been taken far too literally. Cartoon and slapstick comedy plots commonly include...

- Getting hit on the head very hard with an object, but recovering completely and almost instantaneously
- Losing memory and having memory return after a second blow to the head.

Surveys of knowledge about traumatic brain injury have:

- found that the areas of greatest ignorance were about brain injury
- identified how people learn about brain injury
- helped establish priorities
- identified effective public education approaches.

Surveys show that misinformation has a negative impact. As a result, **many people falsely believe...**

- Most people recover from coma or brain injury with no lasting memory or thinking problems.
- Complete recovery from a severe head injury is not possible no matter how motivated the injured person is.
- Everyone can recover if they are motivated enough.
- Recovery is complete once the person with the injury feels "back to normal".
- A second blow to the head can restore memory.
- People can forget who they are and forget other people, but be normal in every other way.
- The harder you work, the faster you recover.
- People with brain injury should rest and remain inactive during recovery.

Recovering and working after brain injury is a tremendous challenge for many. Negative stereotypes make the challenge even greater. Stereotypes about people who are unemployed can be especially painful.

Do Not Be a Victim of Stereotypes... Including Your Own

Try to educate people who stereotype persons with brain injury. Many people have inaccurate beliefs about why individuals with brain injuries are unemployed or underemployed. Encourage others to be understanding and learn the truth.

Believe in the individual rather than the stereotypes of others. Recognize an individual's abilities as well as difficulties. Most individuals...

- Are trying hard to get better and be productive.
- Want to be independent.
- Have at least a few great skills, though other people (sometimes you) may not recognize them.
- Have a lot to contribute.
- Are caring persons with faith and good values.
- Face the same struggles that most people do and are trying to feel good about themselves and their lives.
- Wash their clothes and bathe every day.
- Like it just fine in this country and have the same right as any other citizen to be here.

A person with a brain injury, family members, friends, co-workers, and supervisors may not even recognize that they have negative stereotypes. This tip card has two questionnaires to show the effects of stereotypes. Complete them and review your responses carefully. Think about how you would have answered before your injury or how you would have answered before you knew someone with a brain injury. Do you still hold negative stereotypes? Compare your responses to others who have never met a person with a brain injury.

Talk with friends, family members and coworkers about their responses. Open and honest discussions can help people better understand the effects of a brain injury. Discussion can also help reduce feelings of frustration and isolation that many survivors experience years after their injury.

People Who Do Not Work Questionnaire

Directions: What do people think about people who don't work? Look at the items below and check **T for True** or **F for False** for what you think most people believe.

People who don't work...

Are lazy	☐T	☐F
Would rather live off other people	☐T	☐F
Are dumb	☐T	☐F
Have no place in our society	☐T	☐F
Have no morals or values	☐T	☐F
Could care less about anybody else	☐T	☐F
Are mentally ill	☐T	☐F
Have strange ideas about the value of work	☐T	☐F
Are dirty	☐T	☐F
Should move to another country	☐T	☐F

People With Brain Injury Questionnaire

Directions: What do people think about people who have a brain injury? Look at the items below and check **T for True** or **F for False** for what you think most people believe.

People with a brain injury...

Are retarded	☐T	☐F
Can't take care of themselves	☐T	☐F
Can get out of control at any time	☐T	☐F
Are a burden to society	☐T	☐F
Can't hold a job	☐T	☐F
Are totally different from most people	☐T	☐F
Are mentally ill	☐T	☐F
Don't have feelings	☐T	☐F
Are faking	☐T	☐F
Should live in an institution	☐T	☐F
Recover completely with time	☐T	☐F
Shouldn't go out in public	☐T	☐F

Conclusion

Misunderstandings about people with brain injuries contribute to the challenges and frustrations of getting better. You can't change the beliefs of everyone you know. You can't force everyone you meet to understand. Try to be practical. Spend time with the people who care about you most. Communicate, help them understand, and encourage them to learn more about brain injury and recovery. Show others patience, caring, understanding, and your other good qualities.

Resources

Vet Success
www.vetsuccess.gov

Acknowledgements

Some of this material was adapted, with permission, from: Kreutzer, J. & Kolakowsky-Hayner, S. (1999). *The Brain Injury Workbook: A Guide for Living and Working Productively.* The National Resource Center for Traumatic Brain Injury PO Box 980542, Richmond, VA 23298-0542

Tel: 804-828-9055 www.neuro.pmr.vcu.edu

Thinking about Work
Services That Can Help
Written by: Jeffrey S. Kreutzer, Ph.D., ABPP & Stephanie A. Kolakowsky-Hayner, M.A.

✓ discusses whether to look for work
✓ describes services to prepare for work

Getting Started

After a major illness or injury, many people wonder about work. Some return successfully. Others are convinced they can't work. Some just don't want to work. Many worry about their job skills or limited work experience. Others worry about losing disability benefits if they go to work. A few return to jobs they don't like for less pay. Stress can worsen symptoms and add to uncertainties about the future.

Do any of these people sound familiar?

- I'm not sure what I can do, but I need to do something.
- They offered me minimum wage. Before, I was making $28.
- Wasn't working before, don't want to work now.
- My boss thinks I'm a wreck. If I don't quit, I'll get fired.
- Even though I'm a mess, I have to support my family.
- I've put in fifty applications, but nobody's called me.
- I can keep this job, but I hate it now.

Going back to work may seem very complicated. Finding and getting all the services needed may seem just as complicated. There are a few good ways to start looking for help.

First, contact the people who already know you if you were in a rehabilitation program. Ask them for recommendations and advice. There are many services available through the Veterans Administration (VA) that may be helpful in preparing you to return to employment or in improving your independence and quality of living.

Psychological Services

This involves looking at emotional or mental health before and after becoming disabled. Besides the physical consequences of an illness or injury, there are emotional effects. These may affect a person's interests and abilities to work.

The psychological assessment and referral process may include...

- interviews, reviewing records, and completing questionnaires and tests
- a written report
- reviewing results
- referrals to a counselor, psychologist, or psychiatrist if mental health services are needed.

Social Services

These professionals can identify any special needs for health care, rehabilitation, finances, housing or employment. They also know about eligibility requirements for many programs for persons with disabilities. They can locate community agencies and help with applications by phone contacts, setting up appointments and completing referrals.

The social service professional can help a person with a disability by...

- discussing situations, needs, and goals
- helping with questionnaires
- assisting with eligibility and application forms
- talking with family members and others involved

Transportation Training

A person's ability to drive safely may be affected by a disability. Transportation training can help people with disabilities use public transportation systems or help develop safe driving skills.

The specialist can...

- teach you to read schedules and help you learn when and where to get on and off a bus or subway
- refer you for a driving evaluation
- refer you to a transportation service for persons with special needs

Vocational Services

There are many services through VA's Vocational Rehabilitation and Employment Program (VR&E) that can help an eligible and entitled veteran with choices and decisions about working. But this takes time because every person's needs and abilities are different.

Comprehensive Evaluation

This helps develop an overall picture of a person's interests, abilities, skills, needs, and the likelihood of being successful at work.

The comprehensive evaluation process usually includes...

- reviewing work and academic records
- reviewing treatment records and recommendations
- completing interviews and questionnaires
- testing to measure aptitudes, interests and temperament
- making a referral for a neuropsychological evaluation if there are questions about memory, intellectual, and academic skills
- requesting a referral for a functional capacity evaluation if there are questions about physical endurance and abilities
- identifying other vocational services needed and making referrals.

Vocational Exploration and Counseling

Vocational rehabilitation counselors have special training and experience to help people find work that fits their interests and abilities. It often involves many discussions with the person, family members, and co-workers or supervisors.

The vocational counselor may help a person by...

- discussing needs, interests, and abilities
- developing realistic goals that match abilities, interests and disability requirements
- advising on the rights of a person with a disability
- identifying work related problems and developing solutions or strategies

- identifying needs for other vocational services
- developing a comprehensive plan of services
- giving support throughout the vocational rehabilitation process, including the job search and after being hired

Job Training

The job training process helps develop the skills needed to be productive and efficient on the job.

A vocational rehabilitation counselor or employment coordinator can...

- find books and information
- help plan and organize work
- develop effective compensatory strategies
- arrange for classes or training to improve job skills, if necessary
- set up hands-on experience to learn how to use special tools and equipment

Placement Services

Many people know what kind of job they want, but don't know where to find it.

A vocational rehabilitation counselor or employment coordinator can...

- identify employers with jobs of interest
- talk to employers to learn job requirements
- identify potential safety concerns on the job
- interview potential employers, visit promising work sites, and arrange introductory visits On-Site Support Services

On-site (on the job) support has the advantage of direct contact and observation. A vocational rehabilitation counselor or employment coordinator can arrange face-to-face discussions and training sessions with the person with a disability, the supervisor, and co-workers. It helps to clearly identify any problems as well as strengths on the job.

On-site support services can help a person...

- develop the skills needed for the job
- develop compensatory and organizational strategies to increase efficiency and productivity
- develop a positive attitude and a strong work ethic
- understand and follow rules set by the employer
- communicate and negotiate with an employer and co-workers, sometimes called *job advocacy*
- educate supervisors and co-workers about any disability and special needs

Needs Change Over Time

Most people find that their situation changes over time. Working people may decide to look for another job, cut back on hours, or retire. Unemployed people may decide that the time is right to begin looking for work.

Like many people, your abilities may improve over time. The services that you need will change over time as your hopes, choices, relationships, and finances change. Keeping in touch with the many resources, such as those described here, helps insure that your needs will be met in the long-term. Your patience, persistence and search for information will ultimately lead you to a more productive and satisfying life.

Acknowledgments

Some of this material was adapted, with permission, from: Kreutzer, J. & Kolakowsky-Hayner, S. (1999). *The Brain Injury Workbook: A Guide for Living and Working Productively*.

The National Resource Center for Traumatic Brain Injury

PO Box 980542, Richmond, VA 23298-0542.

Tel: 804-828-9055   www.neuro.pmr.vcu.edu

Resources

Vet Success
www.vetsuccess.gov

The Military Severely Injured Center
www.military.com/support

Back to Work
Options After a Neurological Disability
Written by: Jeffrey S. Kreutzer, Ph.D., ABPP & Stephanie A. Kolakowsky-Hayner, M.A.

✓ identifies challenges for returning to work
✓ describes strategies to work successfully

Want Your Old Job Back?

Any disease, condition or injury that affects the brain can cause physical, mental, emotional, and behavioral changes. Strokes and brain injuries are just two of many conditions that can raise questions about your ability to work again.

A few weeks in the hospital, or even a few weeks at home, can make you miss even the most boring job. You probably miss making money and your friends at work. Maybe your boss, co-workers, or friends have been nagging you to start back right away. You have bills piling up.

No matter how excited you are about working again, going back to the same job may not be the best idea. You may want to think about changing the kind of work you do, who you work for, or your schedule. Maybe you didn't like where you were working in the first place. This is a chance to make a change.

Perhaps you worry about how you'll be treated by supervisors or co-workers. You may be worried about your stamina, headaches, back problems, memory, dizziness, or weakness. These conditions can affect your ability to do the job. There is also the question of safety at work.

Choices

Many people fear going back to their old jobs for many reasons. Fear often stems from worries that supervisors and co-workers will demand the same quality and quantity of work and that you won't be able to keep up. Be careful to avoid making assumptions about what will be expected and how you'll be treated. Most people have more options than they realize. If you look hard enough and long enough, you'll find ways to make your work situation better and increase your chances for success.

The next sections will help you think about returning to your old job and help you identify your options.

Job Safety

Long-term successes start with small, successful steps. Most jobs have easy parts and hard parts. You need to identify both parts. Advice and support from others can help you with the hard parts. Compensatory strategies can also help. The job may need to be set up differently until you are able to do all parts successfully.

Safety is important for every job, but especially now that you have a disability. If you were hurt on the job, you are probably very worried about going back and getting hurt again. The workplace has more risks for people with neurological disabilities than for other workers. What can you do to return to work safely and avoid being injured again?

A job analysis from a vocational rehabilitation counselor can help. The counselor will visit your work site, point out dangers, and make suggestions to improve safety. The counselor may also encourage your supervisor to follow government and company-wide safety regulations. This can create a safer work environment for your co-workers as well.

Understanding how the company you work for has treated people with disabilities in the past may also be helpful. Some employers go out of their way to be supportive. Some offer to be supportive, but don't keep their word. Others ignore or avoid issues relating to disability and job accommodations. Know your rights under the law, especially the Americans with Disabilities Act (ADA). Know the company's personnel policies about hiring, working conditions, job performance, supervision, and grounds for suspension or termination.

Tips on thinking about work...

The following questions will help you think about the work that you want to do, how the workplace is set up, and how you expect to be treated...

✓ What will be hardest for me on the job?

✓ What will be easiest for me on the job?

✓ How will I feel if I can't work as well as before?

✓ Can I change some parts of my job?

✓ Can I change my job but still work at the same place?

✓ Was the workplace safe for me before and has this changed?

✓ Have any of my co-workers been hurt on the job? How?

✓ Are there other people with disabilities working there?

✓ What happened to other people who became ill or disabled after they were hired?

Work Schedule

Fatigue, poor stamina, and pain are very common with a brain disorder. Sleep disturbance is very common. Some people have a hard time falling asleep. Others wake up early and can't get back to sleep. Some wake up many times during the night and don't feel rested in the morning.

Sleep problems and the extra effort required to do even the simplest things cause many persons with brain disorders to feel tired much of the time. Headaches, back pain, and muscle aches are also common. Feeling tired and achy makes it hard to think, be productive, or work a regular schedule.

Most working people with severe disabilities have part-time schedules. When you first start working again, consider starting out part-time. As you succeed, you can build up your hours slowly. Some people have a hard time "getting going" in the morning. Others "fade" in the afternoon. By talking with your supervisor and gearing your schedule to the time of day when you are most energetic, you have a better chance of success.

Scheduling follow-up medical appointments or therapies before or after work may be difficult, especially if you work full-time. Talk with your supervisor about appointments, tests or therapies that are needed and how to best schedule them if you need

time off during the workday. Explain that doing so will help you stay healthier and more productive in the long term.

Tips on scheduling...

To help you think about, organize, and negotiate your work schedule, answer the following questions...

✓ Can I arrange a flexible work schedule?

✓ Will my supervisor let me work part-time?

✓ How will my benefits be affected if I work part-time?

✓ How can I arrange time off for doctor's or therapy appointments?

Supervisors and Co-Workers

Going back to your job after becoming disabled is challenging. It may be harder if you found your job unpleasant or difficult before you became disabled. You may worry that your supervisor won't be patient or helpful. Arrange regular meetings with your supervisor to discuss your progress, strengths, and areas that need improvement. Constructive feedback can be critical to your success. Listening and trying suggestions of supervisors and managers will help convince them that you have a positive attitude and are trying to succeed.

Some supervisors give little or no feedback to any workers. Others avoid giving feedback to workers with disabilities because they are uncomfortable or think that you will take it personally and feel worse. Some employers avoid giving negative feedback because they fear accusations of discrimination by a worker with a disability. Your supervisor's feedback and help are needed for you to succeed. Ask for constructive advice, especially information that emphasizes what you can do to be more successful rather than what you did wrong.

Loneliness and missing the people you work with may be the hardest part of not working after a disability. The support of co-workers after you return to work can be very important to feel accepted and part of a team. You will have many chances to get informal feedback from your co-workers. Seek advice, especially from senior employees and others who do their jobs well.

Tips to improve the feedback process...

✓ Explain how feedback can help you avoid mistakes, failing, and feeling frustrated.

- ✓ Remind people that you want to know about the good things as well as the bad.
- ✓ Be receptive and listen carefully.
- ✓ Make certain that you hear the positive.
- ✓ Show your willingness to change.
- ✓ Avoid defensiveness, "shutting down" and not listening when you hear negative feedback.

To help you think about your co-workers and how they can help you work successfully, answer the following questions...

- ✓ How much did I like the people I worked with before my disability?
- ✓ Will my co-workers accept me if I'm not able to work as well as before?
- ✓ How will my co-workers respond if I need their help in the short-term? In the long term?
- ✓ How can I encourage my co-workers to give me helpful feedback?

Conclusion

After a neurological disability, returning to your old job can be challenging. Talk to your vocational rehabilitation counselor to carefully consider your options and whether you'd really like to return to work. Success will depend on a number of things including the severity of your disability, the nature of challenges in your job, and the support you get from supervisors and co-workers.

Returning to work is a practical option for many people. Most find that the process takes longer than expected. Take your time deciding about your next steps and seek advice from people who care about you.

Acknowledgments

Some of this material was adapted, with permission, from:

Kreutzer, J. & Kolakowsky-Hayner, S. (1999). *The Brain Injury Workbook: A Guide for Living and Working Productively.*

The National Resource Center for Traumatic Brain Injury

PO Box 980542, Richmond, VA 23298-0542

Tel. 804-828-9055. www.neuro.pmr.vcu.edu

Resources

Vet Success
www.vetsuccess.gov

Work

Myths and Facts About Hiring Individuals with Disabilities
Written by: Susan DePompei, M.A. and Vincent Licenziato

✓ discusses getting a job
✓ helps prepare for interviews
✓ explains job accommodations

Can This Person Do The Job?

This is the first question many employers have when someone with a disability applies for a job. With the support of families and professionals - and passage of the Americans with Disabilities Act (ADA) - there are now more people with disabilities working successfully than ever before. However, employers still have many questions that, if left unanswered, can result in *qualified* individuals with disabilities remaining unemployed. Examples of concerns by employers are... How much can I expect if I hire this person? Who will help with any problems at work? Can I let this person go if the job is not being done correctly? What if this person does something that upsets a customer or co-worker?

When people ask questions, they get an accurate picture of what a person with a disability *can do*. Many employers don't realize that people with disabilities can work; they may just do the job *differently*.

The following myths and facts give information to correct common misunderstandings about the abilities and employment potential of individuals with disabilities. With this information, the biggest barrier to employment - attitude - can be changed.

Myth... People with disabilities are not employable.

Fact... The majority of people with disabilities have abilities that make them employable.

Individuals with disabilities are just that - *individuals* with a variety of experiences, qualities, skills, and education. Stereotypes about people with disabilities portray them as being dependent. The truth is that many people, even those with severe disabilities, can be quite independent and are very employable. Many individuals with disabilities are able to work with the same amount of supervision as anyone else.

Myth... It is against the law for an employer to discuss and ask questions about a person's disability.

Fact... An appropriate, job-focused discussion about the person's disability and the needed accommodation is essential if a reasonable accommodation is needed.

If the disability is visible... *and requires an accommodation*, the person with a disability will help the employer by bringing up the subject and explaining what accommodation is needed and how the job will get done.

If the disability is visible... *but does not require an accommodation*, many employers will still have concerns and doubts about how the job will get done and may even assume the person can't do the job. The person with the disability can let the employer know the disability will not interfere with the job and explain how it will get done.

If the disability is not visible... *and requires an accommodation*, the person with a disability may want to wait until a job offer has been made to discuss what is needed.

If the disability is not visible... *and does not require an accommodation*, a discussion is not needed.

Myth... An employer must hire an individual with a disability if the person is qualified to do the job.

Fact... An employer does not have to give preference to an applicant with a disability over other applicants, but must give equal consideration to the applicant with a disability.

The decision to hire someone is based upon who can perform the *essential functions* of the job *with or without* a reasonable accommodation. The decision must be based on factors *unrelated* to the disability such as skill, experience and education.

If two applicants are equally qualified, and one has a disability, the ADA does not say that the job has to go to the applicant with the disability. However, the ADA does state that an employer can not *deny* employment to someone solely based upon that person's disability.

Myth...*Once an employee with a disability is hired, there is no one to help.*

Fact...*Many vocational rehabilitation agencies provide employment training and assistance to both the employee with a disability and the employer.*

Many employers are concerned that they will be "left on their own" to train an employee who may have a difficult time adjusting to, or understanding, a new job. Job trainers or "coaches" can help accommodate someone's specific learning style or provide additional training when necessary. The job coach will work with employees until they can work independently. Since this is done on-site, both the employee and employer gain confidence by knowing that the job "will get done."

Job coaches are most effective when they work with supervisors to complement existing training for new employees. In addition, co-workers receive guidance on working with someone with a disability.

Myth...*People with disabilities work and behave the same way.*

Fact...*People with disabilities are individuals with unique characteristics.*

Even when an employer has had an experience with someone with a disability, it does not mean the next individual, even someone with the same disability, will be anything like the first person. While there may be some common cognitive, physical, or emotional characteristics, *all* people are individuals.

Just because one method of job training worked in the past with someone, it does not mean that it will work with a different individual who has a similar disability. Job trainers and vocational rehabilitation counselors are experienced in working with people on an individualized basis.

Myth...*If an individual with a disability is hired, the employer must fully modify the work environment.*

Fact...*An employer must provide a reasonable accommodation if it is requested.*

An employer must provide a reasonable accommodation for someone to perform the *essential functions* of a job unless the employer can show that the accommodation would cause an *undue hardship*. A reasonable accommodation does not mean that the quality or quantity of work is lowered. It means that a job may be learned or done differently.

An undue hardship means an employer is unable to function at the same level of business. Some reasonable accom- modations include using a telephone headset, adjusting the work schedule, raising a desk, giving written instructions, or installing a ramp.

There is no set criteria for a reasonable accommodation. What is reasonable for one employer may not be reasonable for another. While a large employer may be able to afford an accommodation, that same accommodation may cause an undue hardship for a small business. Reasonable accommodations are made on a case-by-case basis depending upon the job, the individual and the place of employment.

Myth...*Co-workers have to change their jobs to accommodate the work needs of a person with a disability.*

Fact...*A reasonable accommodation is made for the person with the disability and should not affect any other employee.*

Expecting more productivity from other employees to make up for less work by an individual with a disability is not a reasonable accommodation. Productivity goals must be established for all individuals - regardless of disability - without putting unrealistic expectations on others.

Myth...*Employers must accept a lower quality of work because of the employee's disability.*

Fact...*Employees with disabilities must meet the same quality standards.*

All employees working in similar positions must, and should, be held to the same standards of performance. An individual with a disability is not *excused* from producing and completing a job to an employer's satisfaction. The employer should address any difficulties or lower levels of productivity that relate to the disability and, when possible, provide an accommodation.

If accommodations do not improve the quality of work, it may mean that this person is not *qualified* for the job. Problems unrelated to the disability - lack of effort, tardiness, and poor attitude - must, and should, be dealt with by the employer the same way as with any other employee.

Myth... Once an individual with a disability is hired, the employer cannot fire this person.

*Fact... **Employees with disabilities are subject to the same policies and procedures as all other employees.***

Many employers fear the ADA means they will be sued if they fire an individual with a disability. It is important that all employees be treated fairly *and* all employees be held to the same standards. Although the law protects people from being fired *because* of their disability, employers have the right to terminate *any* employee who is not performing satisfactorily, disability or not.

The Bottom Line - Conclusion

During the first several months of employment, it is especially important to continue meeting with your vocational rehabilitation counselor who can help coordinate necessary accommodations, job coaching or other services you need to remain successfully employed. Employment is a large part of many people's lives. Employers take risks everyday when they hire someone. Hiring an individual with a disability may seem like a bigger risk. But individuals with disabilities have abilities and skills to contribute to the success of any business. Employers need to keep this in mind when hiring. Remember, a limitation does not mean inability.

Resources

US Dept of Labor, Office of Disability Employment Policy
www.dol.gov/odep/

The Americans with Disabilities Act
www.eeoc.gov/ada/

US Equal Employment Opportunity Commission
www.eeoc.gov

Vet Success
www.vetsuccess.gov